MAN—
His Origin, History and Destiny

WERNER SCHROEDER

A RELENTLESS QUEST FOR TRUTH

Ascended Master Teaching Foundation
Mount Shasta, California

DEDICATION

This book is dedicated to the Great White Brotherhood for Their continuing efforts in bringing enlightenment to the human race, and especially to the Ascended Masters Saint Germain and El Morya, for obtaining the dispensations that are the basis for this work, and without which there would be no hope for the planet; to Guy W. Ballard and Geraldine Innocenti, their messengers, and to seekers of Light and Truth everywhere.

ACKNOWLEDGMENTS

I would like to express my thanks and gratitude to my first teachers, my aunt and uncle the late Bertha and Walter Rabis, to my second teacher, an eyewitness to many of the dictations given, to my wife, Annette, for her continuous support and for editing this book, and to Personal Word Processing, 5365 Baron Drive, San Jose, CA, 95124 for the kind and professional assistance in typesetting.

About the Book and the Author

Written both from a religious and a historic point of view, this book addresses the basic questions of life such as, "Why am I here?", "What is my purpose?", and "Where am I going? Is there life after death and what happens after I transition from the earth-plane?".

The text starts with the very beginning of man's history, namely the advent of man on Earth, and it ends with a description of future events which will affect every one of us. Written in chronological order, the book includes detailed descriptions of man's activities in the "Garden of Eden," the total age of mankind, as well as details of Lemuria, Atlantis and the unknown life of Jesus and Mary.

Part I is based on information given by Higher Intelligences, called Ascended Masters (Jesus, Mary, Buddha and others). In Part II of the book this data is compared with that of historians. Part III contains predictions about the future, and a suggested plan of action in bringing the plan of the Masters, for a New Golden Age, into fruition. Much of the source material has never before been researched and it has not been available through bookstores.

Werner Schroeder was born and educated in Germany. He studied in Berlin and graduated as a Civil Engineer. After residing in West Germany and Canada, he became a citizen of the United States.

Werner Schroeder qualified as a Registered Civil Engineer in California, and worked for over twenty years as a project engineer and as a project manager, with a specialty in highway design. In January of 1984, he retired and moved with his family to Mount Shasta. Here he intends to do further research.

In 1973 the author became interested in Ascended Master Teaching. This book is the result of his research.

P.O. Box 466, Mount Shasta, CA. 96067

Foreword

It is with a feeling of deep gratitude that I present this book to the reader for his consideration. Much of the information given has never before been published and been available in bookstores. It is data that the Masters of Wisdom were not previously allowed to reveal. Even illumined souls such as Helen Blavatsky, Mary Baker Eddy and Alice Bailey were not privileged to receive such knowledge. Why? — because this type of information, until 1930, was only allowed to be given in the retreats of the Great White Brotherhood, the Brotherhood of Light. Even then there were restrictions. All of the information was given sparingly and gradually, and somewhat veiled. It was up to the student to ponder the message. Only students of a high spiritual development were allowed to enter a retreat. After a certain intermediate stage of retreat-training was reached, a commitment was required of the student to serve the cause of the Brotherhood, and he was initiated.

In the early thirties, this action of Cosmic Law — called Occult Law — was set aside. Ascended Master Teaching may now be given in a simple, straightforward manner. Hiding spiritual truth in legends, fables, myths and parables is no longer required.

I was always a seeker of truth, but it was not until 1973, that something prompted me "that there was more." I started by reading the books *Life and Teaching of the Masters of the Far East*, by Baird Spaulding. After reading the five volumes I wrote to the publisher, inquiring if anybody had done any research on these books, regarding some of the claims made. The answer was negative. I decided to commence with my own research.

In 1976, I had the good fortune of becoming acquainted with a person who had attended Mr. Ballard's lectures and dictations in the 1930's (the "I AM Activity.") In the 1950's she had assisted with recording the messages that the Ascended Masters gave through Geraldine Innocenti. Since this individual prefers to stay in the background, I shall hereafter refer to her as "the eyewitness."

Several years ago, the eyewitness was kind enough to invite my wife and myself to her home, and during a 20 hour interview we were introduced into the fundamentals of Ascended Master Teaching. When confronted with the question of why the public does not know more about the subject, she said of existing organizations, "they that give it out haven't got it straight and they that have it straight won't give it out." This visit established the momentum needed for our future work.

The idea of compiling this book was first perceived about 7 years ago. It was prompted by the following:

1) I became convinced that the messages received through the messengers Guy W. Ballard and Geraldine Innocenti were genuine, and internally consistent. They matched almost perfectly. Considering that in some instances the dictations were given thirty-one years apart, I found this to be rather amazing.
2) For years I had looked for other channels of the Masters, including those living in foreign countries, and compared the testimony to the one I researched. There was simply no comparison. None of the other dictations even closely approached in substance the messages given through Mr. Ballard and G. Innocenti.
3) Anytime I wanted to present some information on

ancient historical events I found myself preparing for many hours. The information on history was scattered among the dozens of monthly publications and books that were the basis for this work. It was like placing together the pieces of a 5000-piece jigsaw puzzle, which, if completed, might contain the most valuable collection of historical data ever offered to mankind since the days of the sinking of Atlantis.

4) I wanted to present to the reader a choice, a choice never before available because the original material was not freely given out. Much of this material has not been published for a long time and few sets of the original material are left in the hands of individuals.

5) I perceived a greater challenge, a greater need, and a greater opportunity, to write a book on history rather than on Cosmic Law. Several good books have been written on Cosmic Law. None that I know of treat the subject of history in detailed, chronological order and base this work on the dictations of the Masters of Wisdom.

6) The understanding of Cosmic Law helps one to understand the significance of historical events. In many instances I was able to show the reader not only what happened, by why it happened.

7) It became clear to me that the testimony of an Ascended Master is very much superior to that of an unascended being having the gift of clairvoyance. Only an Ascended Master can read the Akashic Records correctly. This will become more clear as the reader is acquainted with the testimony of some of the psychics, under the topic "Early Man."

8) I happened to agree with Dr. D. Zink, who stated in his book, *The Stones of Atlantis*, that any significant expansion of our understanding of

prehistory will have a crucial effect upon our present civilization, perhaps even upon its survival.

9) The message of the Ascended Masters contained a strong warning that should concern every individual living on this planet. I wanted people to be aware of the impact of this message. The Masters stated that we are literally sitting on a powder keg and that certain earth changes stand before us that will affect everyone. There is no way that these changes can be avoided, but the loss of property and lives can still be minimized. They also said in the 1950's, "This is the last effort to free mankind." This I interpret to mean, that it would be difficult for the Great White Brotherhood to be granted a new dispensation from the Hierarchy of the system if the original message given in the 1930's and 1950's is not fully utilized. The book contains a plan of action, originally proposed by the Masters, that would, if followed, take full advantage of the original dictations, lessen the impact of the earth changes and bring in a Permanent Golden Age.

Obtaining the original messages proved rather difficult and time-consuming, but if one is sincere and persistent, the Great Cosmic Law will provide. After nearly two years of effort, we received practically all of the original information given through the two channels. The parents of two students had been part of the original effort. We received two packages. When we opened them, the material fitted together perfectly. What was missing from one package, was contained in the other. This was the first proof we were on the right track.

If there were any doubts about my writing this book, these doubts were completely removed through some experiences I had on Mount Shasta. It was here, at a place where I believe Mr. Ballard first met Saint Germain, that I received the confirmation I was looking for. The way this happened will always be remembered.

Now the referencing and cataloguing started in earnest. Thousands of reference cards were prepared. The original material, if placed together, probably could fill one book, 6 inches by 9 inches by 60 inches thick. The reader can rest assured that all of the material on the subject of history that was ever given through the two messengers mentioned, is shown in this book. However, if a student has additional information, I would appreciate knowing about it.

The story of this book reminds me of our last trip to the European Alps. One never knew what to expect; after nearly every turn there were new vistas, new fields to explore.

As far as the source material for this work is concerned, with few exceptions, I found it to be relatively easy to analyze. The dictations, for the most part, were written in a simple, straightforward manner. An exception to this, I believe, are some of the dictations on the formation of our galaxy. I did not find any student that could help me with this. It took months of reading and re-reading the material before I was able to present to the reader what I believe the Masters were trying to say. The key to this were some dictations that did not deal specifically with the subject.

According to Cosmic Law, I have to account for every word written in this book. Thus, absolute accuracy and congruency with the original text was considered of prime importance. Also, no attempt was made to make the information given by the Masters fit with existing theories or standards. For example, the life history of Jesus and Mary is strictly based on original dictations; the *Bible* was not used for reference.

Let me explain briefly what an Ascended Master is.

In simple terms, it is an individual who once was embodied here on Earth, but gained mastery of this plane. He learned his lesson, became more God-like, and therefore did not have to come back into embodiment. Then, after having ascended into his spiritual body, called the I AM Presence, the Master made the voluntary choice to postpone his further development; he chose to remain and help mankind.

The Ascended Masters are REAL and TANGIBLE BEINGS, ready to assist mankind, provided they are asked to do so. Among the Masters more known are Jesus, Mary, Moses, Saint Germain, Gautama Buddha and Lord Krishna. They are part of a group of Avatars (world teachers) who since the fall of man have carried the word of God for the enlightenment of the human race. The Masters ask to be recognized as a potential force for the common good of mankind, but They do not demand obedience and do not ask to be worshipped.

The Great White Brotherhood is not an outer organization. Only by living and expressing the perfection of the heavenly realm on the physical plane, through self-correction of human weaknesses and full adoration of the Divine Self within, can an individual draw himself into association with the Brotherhood. The Ascended Host directs the attention of the chela, but it is up to the student to make the right choices. No individual ever made the ascension without the assistance of an Ascended Master.

The Hierarchy of the Earth consists of Ascended Beings. Its structure may be compared to that of a business such as General Motors; there is always another level of supervision. The Ascended Masters are the Directing Intelligence of the Godhead; They are God's helpers. It is that simple.

Some may question as to how it is possible for an Ascended Being to contact an individual on the physical plane and get a clear message through. That is a more difficult question which will be answered in the text of this book. Here, I would like to say this. It is recognized by orthodox churches that Jesus had unlimited power. If this is so, why is it so improbable that He can contact a humble, sincere, spiritually-enlightened individual? If one is looking for proof, perhaps it should be mentioned that 20,000 instantaneous healings have been attributed to Mr. Ballard's work over a period of five years. There is no greater proof needed.

Ascended Master Teaching is a harmonious blend of Western and Eastern teachings. It complements the consciousness of the Orient (which is predominantly worship without sufficient works) with the vital energies of the Western consciousness (which is predominantly works without sufficient worship). It is the teaching that was originally recorded in the New Testament. Later, according to the Masters, the *Bible* suffered through many translations and was embellished by personal imprints. The Masters stated that Genesis and all of the succeeding Biblical chapters needed to be re-written. This time the text was written by Ascended Beings.

Ascended Master Teaching stands on its own, and is neither Christian, Moslem, Jewish or Hindu. It may be called the root, the Fountain of Truth, from which all known religions had their source.

This book will never be complete. The quest must continue as long as **one** facet of man's ancient history, from which a lesson can be learned, remains uncovered. Much has been given, much remains to be done. May there be students who will wish to complete this book.

Not everybody will be convinced by the message contained in this publication. Undoubtably it will be attacked. Some leaders of orthodox, established thought, both in the field of religion and science, will attempt to ridicule and criticize portions of it, never offering an overall constructive solution. Recently one modern scientist did just that, hammering away at some point of an overall theory. When the audience asked him for an overall evaluation, he hesitated and said, "Fortunately, I don't have to explain it."

William James, a pioneer psychologist, stated, "Any new theory first is attacked as absurd; then is admitted to be true, but obvious and insignificant; finally it seems to be important, so important that its adversaries claim they themselves discovered it."

To the sincere student, public criticism of this message does not matter. He will know the truth, by calling his I AM Presence into action and by pondering the message in his heart.

The sole purpose of this book is to present for mankind's enlightenment certain information received from the Ascended Masters in the 1930's and 1950's — information which will be seen to apply to today's conditions. I believe the Ascended Masters will watch closely what happens from here on; this may be the first time in this century that somebody has written a book on this subject in such detail. I think their main interest will not be in how many books are sold, but in what individuals will do with the information given. Will it go back on some shelf the same way as other books, or will it stir some feeling and bring about a change in attitude and behavior?

In presenting this message of the Masters, it is my sincere hope and prayer that the reader may receive the "Light" and be blessed and prosper as he walks along the path of enlightenment and service, for by this path, alone, can permanent happiness be found.

It was on Mount Shasta that Saint Germain's effort started, and it was on this holy mountain that I wrote a portion of this foreword. From this vicinity the effort will be continued.

Easter, 1984 Werner Schroeder

CONTENTS

PART I

MAN, HIS ORIGIN AND HIS HISTORY - AS TOLD BY THE GREAT WHITE BROTHERHOOD

1 — CREATION

2 — THE FIRST TWO GOLDEN AGES - THE GARDEN OF EDEN

3 — THE FALL OF MAN

4 — THE AGE OF MAN

5 — SANAT KUMARA SAVES THE EARTH

6 — THE LEMURIAN AGE
(4,500,000 B.C.? to 200,000 B.C.)

7 — THE ATLANTEAN AGE
(500,000 B.C. to 10,000 B.C.)

8 — THE TIME PERIOD FROM POSEIDONIS TO JESUS

9 — THE LIFE OF JESUS AND MARY

10 — THE TIME PERIOD FROM JESUS TO 1961

PART II

ATLANTIS VERIFIED

1 — PLATO´S DIALOGUES

2 — OTHER EVIDENCE FOR ATLANTIS

PART III

MAN'S DESTINY

1 — PREDICTIONS

2 — LEADERSHIP

3 — VISIONS OF A GOLDEN AGE

PART I
MAN, HIS ORIGIN AND HIS HISTORY — AS TOLD BY THE GREAT WHITE BROTHERHOOD

1 - Creation

THE NATURE OF GOD

"So God created man in his own image, in the image of God created He him; male and female created He them." (Genesis 1:27)

The very nature of God, Light, is to expand perfection. Out of love, God gave intelligent consciousness to life, so that man and other forms of life could share the joy of His creation.

All creation consists of perfected forms, accompanied by harmonious sound. Cosmic creation takes place to a symphony of exquisite melody. Every individual sent forth from the heart of the Creator has a particular note or tone, which is established by a consciously-created wave length. That cosmic tone, emitted by every electron of that particular lifestream, flows out continually as a part of the "music of the spheres." As the electrons swing around the central core of Love, their speed determines the note which may be used in any number of blends, and this creation is a cosmic harmony of sounds.

Each electron, containing within itself the fire of

creation, may become the nucleus or cause of whatever form the individual decrees into existence. Therefore, an electron may become the body of a child, the seed of a spiritual idea, the heart of a novel, or a celestial symphony.

Every solar system is governed by a pair of perfected beings, one masculine, and one feminine. Helios and Vesta are the intelligences who are leading the solar system of which our Earth is part.

Love is the key. Through love, Helios and Vesta, projected forth every planet at just the right distance. Through love, every galaxy is held within its orbit around a central focus as it rushes through space with lightning-like speed toward a destiny known only by the Godhead. Similarly, the love and radiation of a sun to its planets causes each one to rotate on its own axis and move in orderly procession around it. This action is part of a glorious train of light made up of millions of galaxies that move by Cosmic Intelligence, whose consciousness is beyond description. All move in precision around a Central Focus, which may be called the Godhead.

Man's reason for being, then, is to become a conscious co-creator with God, to draw life's energy, to take some of the ideas of the Father, plant them in his consciousness, mold them into form, and bring them into fruition on the physical realm, thereby expanding the borders of God-consciousness.

Creation on the physical plane is more difficult than creation on realms of a higher vibratory level. Therefore, individuals which select this experience will be able to do more upon completing the schoolroom of the Earth. The goal is to achieve mastery over energy and vibration and to become more God-like. If man achieves this goal, he will be able to do higher tasks. He may become a member of the Intelligences which jointly govern a planet or he may even create a planet, a sun, yes an entire galaxy.

OUR GALAXY

Introduction

Understanding the fundamental laws underlying the origin and end of a galaxy is not as difficult as one might think.

All creation follows Cosmic Law and a precisely pre-determined general pattern. There is no natural selection by chance or random as some natural scientists lead us to believe. Within this pattern of creation, each individual can exercise his freedom of choice. Each component of a galaxy, therefore, evolves on a pattern of life, which is a succession of experiences, governed by free will. The purpose of a galaxy is, then, to give various forms of life opportunity for individual growth.

Components of a Galaxy

Planet:	A planet serves to give different forms of life, namely mankind, angels and elemental life of the four elements (air, earth, fire, water) opportunity for self-expression and growth. Each planet is governed by several intelligences, which administer Cosmic Law as it applies to the planet.
Sun:	A sun is the life-giving and life-

sustaining element of a solar system, containing itself and several planets. Each sun is governed by two intelligences, one male and one female. Our sun (focus of the Solar Lords Helios and Vesta) is fourth in distance from the Central Sun of our galaxy.

Central Sun: The Central Sun is the focus of the Godhead in a galaxy. It is the owner and giver of all life and of all things within it. It may be considered the sun behind our physical sun. Our Central Sun is the focus of the Divine Beings Alpha and Omega. For our present limited consciousness, this is as close as we can come in understanding the nature of God.

Galaxy: A galaxy consists of the Central Sun and several solar systems. Our particular galaxy consists of seven solar systems, each solar system in turn consists of one sun and seven planets. Therefore, our galaxy consists of the Central sun, seven suns and 49 planets. Some galaxies have thousands of planets. Galaxies are in constant motion and move in a spiral.

The Divine Plan for our Galaxy

An understanding of the Rhythmic Breath is essential to grasp how a galaxy is formed and how it ends. The Rhythmic Breath is a natural activity of Life.

This activity consists of four basic steps, as follows:

1) Inbreathing
2) Pause, also called absorbing the breath
3) Breathing out, also called expansion of breath
4) Pause, also called projection of the breath.

At steps 1 and 2, magnetization occurs. At steps 3 and 4 radiation takes place.

On the Outbreath (step 3), the Central Sun breathes forth first the suns and then these suns in turn bring forth their planets into their pre-designated orbital positions.

During the pause (step 4), individual life (that of mankind, angels and elementals) is given the opportunity to develop and fulfill its divine plan.

After this has been accomplished, the Inbreath takes place. The Inbreath occurs in reverse order of the Outbreath. First each sun magnetizes (draws in) its planets. Then the Central Sun absorbs the suns, together with the planets.

The breath at the cosmic level is therefore similar to the breath we take on the physical level. Right now our breath is only a two-step process. We breathe in and we breathe out. Originally, when mankind first came to Earth, man utilized the rhythmic breath, which includes a pause between each inbreath and outbreath.

It should be emphasized, when planets are returned to the aura of the sun or the Central Sun, the individualized beings, such as mankind, continue to exist. They are very comfortable. There is no need to fear the Sun; it is as cool and as refreshing as a mountain breeze. It is not hot as scientists think. It is only as the sun's currents of energy pass through the ether belt of the Earth that they manifest heat. The Sun is the electronic pole; the Earth is the magnetic pole. The ether belt is the element through which the currents are diversified.

There are millions of suns in the universe, all with their own planets circling around them, differing in number and size, but all following the same pattern of rhythm, of harmony, and of ever-expanding perfection.

The Formation of our Galaxy

The formation of our galaxy occurred on the Outbreath. The Outbreath is subdivided into two parts. During part 1 the seven suns take their place in the galaxy and during part 2 the planets of each sun take their position. Each part is subdivided into seven individual steps, as follows (see Fig. 1).

Part 1:

The seven steps of the Outbreath are first performed by the Central Sun. At each step a new Sun is breathed forth. This is accomplished in a vertically descending order until all suns have reached their pre-designated positions. For example, at step one Sun No. 7 is breathed out first, at step two Sun No. 7 moves to the second position and Sun No. 6 moves into the first position. This sequence is repeated until at the last step Sun No. 7 is farthest away from the Central Sun.

Part 2:

Now it is up to the individual suns to perform the function of the Outbreath. This part of the Outbreath is done in horizontal order; it is also done in seven steps. Thus, at step one, the first sun (in reference to distance from the Central Sun) breathes forth its planet No. 7; at the same time Sun No. 2 breathes out is planet No. 7 and the remaining suns do likewise.

At step two, Sun No. 1 moves its planet No. 7 into

the second orbital position (in reference to distance from the sun) and planet No. 6 into the first orbital position. Simultaneously, the remaining six suns perform the same operation as Sun No. 1.

This procedure is followed until all of the 49 planets have assumed their final orbital positions. The Outbreath is now completed, and orbiting around each sun commences.

The next basic step after the Outbreath is called a Pause. It is the purpose of the Pause to give individualizations, namely mankind, elementals and angels, opportunity for self-expression and development on a planet.

Here again the number seven assumes prime importance. In order to be prepared for embodiment, each individual has to go through the schoolroom and gain experience by going through seven spheres, where he gains knowledge and mastery necessary for life on a planet. Thereafter mankind is divided into seven rootraces. Once taking embodiment in the physical realm, everyone must experience the beneficial influence of seven rays in order to gain the ascension. An individual gains the ascension when he has achieved mastery over energy and vibration. This accomplishment frees him from the wheel of birth and re-birth. The subject of "Spheres," "Rootraces," "Rays" and "Cycles" will be treated in more detail elsewhere in this book.

The time period of the Pause, or the holding of the Outbreath for this galaxy, was to be about 98,000 years. This period of time is needed to give all of the seven rootraces the opportunity to make the ascension. Each rootrace was to gain the ascension in 14,000 years. It takes the beneficial radiation of seven rays (each ray having a duration of 2,000 years) for each member of a rootrace to make the ascension. There is some overlap in the coming-in of rootraces, therefore the number of 98,000 years is only an approximation. After 98,000 years the Inbreath was to start. As all of us know, the perfection of the Earth is far from complete. Billions of lifestreams have not gained their ascension. Since perfection has been maintained on the other planets of our galaxy, the Earth is holding up the divine plan for the entire galaxy.

The End of our Galaxy

The seven steps of the Inbreath occur in opposite order of the Outbreath. As we recall, during the last step of the Outbreath, all planets moved to their final position, and thereby the planet Mercury, together with the six other planets of the other six suns, moved from the aura of their respective suns to orbital position No. 1.

Those planets which were breathed out last, namely Mercury and the other six planets of vertical column No. 1 on the first step of the Inbreath, will be first to move back to the aura of their respective suns. At the same time the other vertical rows of planets will also move one step closer to the seven suns.

The same procedure will be followed during the following six steps, until all of the vertical rows of planets have returned to their suns. Finally, the suns, ascending vertically after completing the seven steps of the Inbreath of the Central Sun, will return to the electronic belt of the Central Sun. This belt is of tremendous size.

After the completion of the Inbreath, a council

will be held, and a decision will be made, again by free will, determining whether suns such as Helios and Vesta wish to become Central Suns, and planets such as the Earth wish to become suns.

The above description tells of the underlying principles that govern the divine plan for our galaxy. Since Cosmic Law is precise, impartial, and uniform in its application, it may be safely assumed that the same procedures apply also to other galaxies. The Masters of Wisdom explained the formation of the galaxy that was the predecessor of our galaxy. The principles used for the formation of that galaxy were exactly identical to the ones just given for our galaxy, and will now be described.

Our Parent Galaxy

The Ascended Masters not only explained the formation of our galaxy, but also gave us details as to the origin of our galaxy. This way we are able to trace the earlier path of evolution of our God-parents Helios and Vesta, as well as that of our Central Sun, which is governed by Alpha and Omega. This investigation also explains the origin of the numbers seven and twelve, that have such a determining influence on our galaxy, on our solar system — yes, on our very lives.

According to a dictation by the Goddess Vesta, our present galaxy evolved from a former galaxy, headed by two Divine Beings, most closely spelled in English as Elohae and Eloha. Elohae represented the masculine aspect, and Eloha, the feminine. This former galaxy consisted of 12 suns, and each sun in turn was responsible for twelve planets (see Fig. 2).

		Orbital position of planets						
	CS **(A)	#1	#2	#3	#4	#5	#6	#7
	*1	.	.	.	.	.	.	.
	*2	.	.	.	.	.	.	.
	*3	.	.	.	.	.	.	.
Suns	*4(H)	M	.	.	E	.	.	.
	*5	.	.	.	.	.	.	.
	*6	.	.	.	.	.	.	.
	*7	.	.	.	.	.	.	.

Fig. 1 – Our Galaxy

H = Helios & Vesta, M = Mercury, E = Earth,
CS = Central Sun, A = Alpha & Omega

		Orbital position of planets											
	**CS	#1	#2	#3	#4	#5	#6	#7	#8	#9	#10	#11	#12
	*1	.	.	.	.	.	.	.	.	.	.	.	.
	*2	.	.	.	.	.	.	.	.	.	.	.	.
	*3	.	.	.	.	.	.	.	.	.	.	.	.
	*4(A)	.	.	.	H	.	.	.	.	.	.	.	.
Suns	*5	.	.	.	.	.	.	.	.	.	.	.	.
	*6	.	.	.	.	.	.	.	.	.	.	.	.
	*7	.	.	.	.	.	.	.	.	.	.	.	.
	*8	.	.	.	.	.	.	.	.	.	.	.	.
	*9	.	.	.	.	.	.	.	.	.	.	.	.
	*10	.	.	.	.	.	.	.	.	.	.	.	.
	*11	.	.	.	.	.	.	.	.	.	.	.	.
	*12	.	.	.	.	.	.	.	.	.	.	.	.

Fig. 2 – Our Parent Galaxy

Our present Central Sun (governed by Alpha and Omega), was part of that galaxy. It was the fourth sun, relative in distance from the Central Sun.

Our present Sun (the focus of Helios and Vesta) was also part of that former galaxy; it was the fourth planet relative in distance from the Sun governed by Alpha and Omega.

The former galaxy completed its divine plan. All of mankind ascended and all planets were absorbed into the aura (electronic belt) of Elohae and Eloha.

Each of the intelligences responsible for a Central Sun, a sun, or planet then decided how they wanted to progress.

Seven of the twelve suns decided to become Central Suns. Alpha and Omega were among these. They became responsible for a galaxy consisting of seven suns, each sun having seven planets.

The choice of these seven suns to become Central Suns established the number seven as the governing number for the galaxy of which we are part.

The total number of suns also impressed a mark upon our galaxy. The Zodiac of each of the suns of our galaxy consists of twelve signs, each expressing one God-virtue, and radiating that quality for about 30 days from the Sun to the planets. The number of keys in an octave on a piano, counting both black and white, is twelve. The seven white keys represent the seven suns who elected to, and were found qualified to, become Central Suns. The five black keys stand for the five suns who did not accomplish this goal. All individualizations of the former galaxy, Helios and Vesta included, have a causal body consisting of 12 concentric bands. All individuals belonging to the galaxy of which the Earth is part, have a causal body consisting of seven concentric bands.

Helios and Vesta made the choice of progressing, and thus took initiation as a sun which was to be responsible for a solar system consisting of a sun and seven planets, including our Earth.

The Ascended Masters gave additional information about life on other planets. They also gave the names of the 49 planets of our galaxy, and included some explanation as to why the names of the planets of our solar system do not fully correspond with those given by natural scientists.

THE CREATION OF OUR EARTH

Introduction

"As above, so below," is a well-known expression. Every physical manifestation is preceded by some action at higher, inner levels.

The Earth was not created in six days — six twenty-four hour periods — as stated in the Bible. It manifested over a long period of time, as a result of a series of decisions and actions involving mainly the seven Creators of our solar system. These Creators are called the Elohim.

After Helios and Vesta decided to become God Father and Mother of our solar system, they had to prove, through the directing of light rays, that they could radiate enough concentrated energy to first create a solar system, then to maintain its planets in a certain orbital position, and to sustain life thereon. Helios and Vesta passed the initiation; thus Alpha and Omega vested them with the authority for such a system.

The first fiat issued by Helios and Vesta was, "Let there be Light." Through thought and feeling Helios and Vesta determined the size of the planets, their location, and the number of lifestreams that would abide on each one. This could be compared to our designing of a home and the interiors that go with it.

When the light pattern was completed, Helios and Vesta placed the blueprint into the hands of the Cosmic Silent Watcher, who is responsible for holding the pattern of our galaxy. The name of the Cosmic Silent Watcher is Serculata, a feminine being.

Serculata absorbed the pattern of design, and accepted the responsibility of holding the immaculate concept for each planet until the time when Helios and Vesta would designate the externalization of each. The blueprint contained the oceans, seas, rivers, lakes, lands, trees, shrubs and other vegetation, the mountains and atmosphere for each planet.

When the time for the creation of the Earth was at hand, the Cosmic Silent Watcher turned the blueprint over to its Planetary Silent Watcher. The name of the Earth's Silent Watcher is Immaculata, also a feminine being.

Now Helios and Vesta drew forth the seven Elohim, and the Devas who would be directing the Builders of Form. Meeting regularly at specific time intervals, together they started to manifest the Earth into physical form, using the light pattern given by the Planetary Silent Watcher, and using the standard system for the creation of a planet, a process called "the seven steps to precipitation."

The Seven Steps to Precipitation

All planets are created using the Law of Precipitation. Precipitation, as used in this book, means to manifest a material thing out of primary, electronic, light substance. An example of precipitation is Jesus' feeding of the five thousand, as recorded in the Scriptures.

The Law of Precipitation was used during the Golden Ages, which the Earth was to enjoy at a later time. Since Cosmic Law does not change, it applies as well today, and any student may use it to his advantage in his daily affairs.

In order to understand how the Law of Precipitation operates, it is important to first learn about the action of the seven rays. Following here are the general characteristics of each ray, and an example is given as to how each ray was used in the specific case of creating the Earth.

General action and characteristics of the First Ray (color blue): the WILL, power, and determination to make a decision. Without the will to do something, there is no accomplishment. Before making a decision, one should use prayerful thought and investigate one's motive.

Specific case: Hercules, the Elohim of the First Ray, as spokesman for the seven Elohim, said to Helios and Vesta, "We WILL externalize your pattern and plan."

Second Ray (yellow): PERCEPTION (illumination) to recognize the idea, to grasp it, to draw forth the ways and means enabling quick and permanent manifestation.

Specific case: Elohim Cassiopea helped to PERCEIVE the glory of each planet as Helios and Vesta intended, including the mountains, the rivers and the valleys.

Third Ray (pink): DIVINE LOVE, the power of cohesion, draws the unformed into form. Love draws primal life (electrons) and makes it available to be placed into a lower vibratory level. This light-substance then obediently takes manifest form according to the pattern previously perceived. Love is a necessary ingredient during each step of an endeavor until it is completed. The more sincere feelings of love one can put into a desired manifestation, the more beautiful will be the form, and the more quickly it will manifest.

If love would cease to be, all of the universe would return to the unformed. For example, deserts are places where elementals refuse to bring forth plant life.

Specific case: It was LOVE that made the Seven Elohim say, "We will take part in the creation of the planets, accepting the design of Helios and Vesta, rather than our own." Elohim Orion brought forth the Flame of Divine Love, that drew out of universal substance the necessary ingredients to eternalize the globe according to the design of Helios and Vesta.

Fourth Ray (white): PURITY is a matter of feeling, of consciousness, holding steady the picture, keeping it pure, not distorting it by any opinion or desire of the outer self. Through the Flame of Purity the original idea is perfected in its finest detail and clarity.

Specific case: Claire, the Elohim of the Fourth Ray, held inviolate the original design of Helios and Vesta, so that not one mountain, one tree, nor even a blade of grass would manifest out of his own design.

Fifth Ray (green): CONCENTRATION and CONSECRATION. Concentration must rest upon the original idea or light pattern, adding energy through feeling and consecration of the individual to the task at hand, until the form is totally completed — the "stick-to-it-iveness." If one is able to concentrate upon one thing at a time, one is able to produce a manifestation. If there is no concentration, there is only mediocrity. Without concentration the once-desired manifestation is abandoned before it actually appears. The "invisible realm" is filled with incomplete prayers, with beautiful thought-forms that were sometimes within ONE hour of expression.

Being "jack of all trades but master of none" should not be one's ultimate goal. Determination is needed to rise above the masses. Take ONE facet of living, masterfully develop it, and excel at least along ONE line.

The Elohim of the Fifth Ray, Vista, said in a dictation: "CONCENTRATION AND CONSECRATION ARE ALMOST THE SAME BECAUSE FIRST OF ALL, WHATEVER YOU ARE GOING TO DO THAT WILL AMOUNT TO ANYTHING REQUIRES THE CONSECRATION OF YOUR LIFE."

Specific case: The concentration of energy by Elohim Vista enabled angels and elementals, including the Builders of Form, to coalesce primal life substance, drawing the Earth into form.

Seventh Ray (violet) — (for purposes of precipitation the order of the sixth and seventh ray are reversed): RHYTHM. Through the use of the Violet Fire and rhythm of invocation, the form receives its finishing touches; it is filed and polished to obtain perfect symmetry, beauty, and general perfection. Rhythm is necessary to provide substance to the form; for example, in our physical body the rhythm of the heartbeat and that of the breath determine the efficiency of our physical form.

Specific case: Arcturus, Elohim of the Seventh Ray, through RHYTHM OF INVOCATION, planed, polished and perfected the Earth until it sparkled like a many-faceted diamond.

Sixth Ray (ruby or gold): PEACE. Sealing the completed manifestation within the flame of Cosmic Christ Peace is an action of the Sixth Ray. This enables the creation to be permanently sustained. Where harmony and peace abide, that which has been drawn forth cannot disintegrate.

Specific case: Tranquility, the Elohim of the Sixth Ray set the completed Earth in motion around its axis, enfolding it in his mantle of peace, sustaining the form permanently. This axis is a current of energy, a light ray from the North Pole to the South Pole. Now the Earth assumed its rightful place among the planets of the galaxy, joining triumphantly in the celestial song of the Music of the Spheres.

THE CREATION OF MAN

Creation of the I AM Presence

After the Seven Elohim and the lesser builders of form (the devas and elementals) created and beautified the planet, Helios and Vesta drew from the Central Sun billions of spirit sparks. A spirit spark may be defined as primal intelligence, having a causal body, white in color, and needing the love of a Solar Lord, in this case Helios and Vesta, for further expression.

While these spirit sparks rested for some time in their vicinity, the God Parents projected light rays from their hearts. These rays converged and formed individual three-fold flames of God-Consciousness. Utilizing these flames as magnets for drawing universal light-substance, Helios and Vesta then created individually-designed garments for the spirit sparks. These bodies of light are called Electronic Bodies.

When this was accomplished, each spirit spark was transferred by Helios and Vesta into the flame within the heart of an Electronic Body. This action results in a White Fire Being, also called an Electronic Presence. It is conscious of its identity, and through the words "I AM," finds itself a living, breathing intelligence, vested with life, opportunity, and free will.

Now the White Fire Being must decide whether or not to voluntarily project the Dual Aspect (masculine and feminine), of its divine nature. Those choosing to go on out further project forth two rays, called "Twin Rays." At the end of each ray is a Threefold Flame, around which is drawn light substance, forming the Electronic Body of the I AM Presence. These I AM Presences have a Causal Body, white in color. (Causal Bodies are discussed under "Seven Bodies of Man.") The I AM Presences are now prepared for embodiment by entering a schoolroom. This preparation is called the "Journey through the Seven Spheres."

Journey Through the Seven Spheres

The individual I AM Presences, each at its own pace, then begin the journey through the seven inner spheres, which are seven concentric bands of color around our sun. Here contact is made with highly-developed intelligences which express the particular qualities of each sphere. These God-Intelligences are desirous of doing the Father's will, expanding His kingdom and consciousness.

Starting with the first sphere, the individual lifestreams (I AM Presences) have the opportunity to absorb the qualities of each sphere, abiding in each as long as they wish, adding the color of the sphere to their causal bodies as they progress. Typically, an individual is attracted to the properties of one particular sphere, preferring to stay there longer while absorbing its qualities. This preference for one particular sphere often results in the pursuit later, when embodied, of a line of work that closely identifies with the properties prevailing in this sphere.

When an individual stays longer in one sphere and

thus absorbs its qualities more than any other one, then this particular sphere becomes his predominant "sphere of development." In some other literature and present usage, the term "ray" is substituted for "sphere"; therefore, "sphere of development" now becomes "ray of development," or simply "he/she is on the second ray."

While the properties of a sphere and a ray are similar, their functions are different. A ray is part of a cycle. A cycle lasts 14,000 years, and is made up of seven rays, each lasting 2,000 years. Therefore all of us experienced many times the beneficial influence of a ray, but only once went through the seven spheres.

The experiences gained while dwelling in a particular sphere may be likened to going to school before embodiment on a planet.

As in other experiences of life, free will is involved, and most of the individuals elect to stay in one of seven spheres. Only one of every twelve White Fire Beings progresses to embodiment. The others elect to stay somewhere along the path, preferring to work there at inner levels.

The following is a summary of the colors and qualities of each sphere. Also shown are corresponding occupations that an individual may have while embodied at a later time, expressing the qualities of that ray. Treating this subject in greater detail is considered beyond the scope of this book.

Sphere	Color	Quality	Service on Planet
1	Blue	Power & Initiative All God-Ideas are born here	Rulers, Leaders & Executives
2	Yellow	Perception, Illumination. Ideas are perceived and moulded into thought patterns and workable form	Educators, Teachers
3	Pink	Love, Tolerance. Ideas are clothed with life essence through the feeling nature, enabling future externalization in the world of form. Love is shown as the cohesive force holding together a manifested form	Peacemakers, Arbitrators
4	Crystal, White	Artistic development. Poetry. Sculpture, Painting	Artists, Musicians, Architects and Poets
5	Green	Scientific Development, Healing, Concentration, Consecration, Truth	Scientists, Engineers, Inventors, Healers, Doctors, and Nurses
6	Ruby, Gold	Devotional Worship	Ministers, Religious Leaders, Missionaries
7	Violet	Culture, Ceremony, Refinement, Diplomacy	Diplomats, Gentlemen

Rootraces, Rays and Cycles

After the I AM Presence has passed through the seven spheres, it is ready to embody on a planet. Each individual presence is assigned a rootrace. This is done by the Manu. It is the function of the Manu to separate those individuals desiring embodiment into seven rootraces and to guard one particular rootrace during its embodiment until each member has made his ascension.

The selection of the members of a rootrace becomes a completely impersonal service. The following factors are considered:

1) The momentum the individual acquired while dwelling in the seven spheres.

This momentum is manifested in the causal body. The causal body has seven concentric bands of color. The width and radiance of the bands tells the Manu about the predominant qualities of the individual. The greater the width of a band, the longer the individual stayed in the sphere corresponding to that particular band.

2) The date when the individual graduated from the seven spheres, thereby completing Earth's schoolroom.

The earlier an individual leaves the seven spheres, the greater are his chances of being part of the first or second rootraces.

3) The circumstance and the conditions where he can be utilized to bless the Earth most.

Individuals of the first sphere (blue) are normally given the chance to embody first, since they provide the anchorage and protection for the entire rootrace. Therefore, the first subrace of a rootrace encompasses, for the most part, individuals predominantly expressing the qualities of the first sphere; however, other individuals not "of the first sphere" are included for added balance. Individuals predominantly "of the second sphere" follow, and so on, until all seven subraces of a particular rootrace are embodied.

As part of the selection process, individuals line up in groups of three. One of each group of three is chosen; the other two remain for future consideration. At some future time they line up in groups of three again.

4) Three and a half billion lifestreams originally chose embodiment on Earth. This number later increased dramatically when individuals from another planet or other planets were allowed to make the Earth their home.

Now let us briefly summarize the functions of rootraces, rays, and cycles, and discuss how they relate to each other.

All individuals seeking embodiment on earth are divided into seven rootraces. Each rootrace in turn consists of seven subraces.

A ray projected from the Central Sun contains the qualities (or God-virtues) of a sphere. The colors and virtues of each sphere were discussed previously. The function of a ray is to nourish one of the seven spiritual centers (chakras). The duration of each ray is 2,000 years, and the number of rays is identical to the number of spheres, namely seven.

The sum of the alternate playing of each of the seven rays upon the Earth is called a cycle. Therefore, a cycle lasts for 14,000 years.

The divine plan for the Earth was to have each member of a rootrace exposed to the alternate playing of seven rays. This would enable each individual to make the ascension. Therefore, the plan called for the first subrace of the first rootrace to make the ascension in 14,000 years. The same plan applied for any other subrace, and each subrace was to enter in intervals of 2,000 years. Since there are 7 rootraces, each rootrace having 7 subraces, we can state that conceptually it should have taken about 100,000 years for all life on Earth to gain the ascension. We all know that this has not taken place. Conditions on the Earth after the "fall of man" have been far from perfect, and billions have not gained the ascension. There are still members of the fourth rootrace with us, who need to balance their karma. However, the first three rootraces and all of their subraces embodied during the first two Golden Ages, and all of them gained their ascension in their allotted time of 14,000 years each. One dictation has stated that the third rootrace took a little longer to gain the ascension, but accomplished it successfully.

The ascension may be considered as methodical as the operation of our present-day gasoline engine. It is a result of consistent application of Cosmic Law. There is no such thing as a miracle. Anyone who knows the Law, applies it, and is persistent in his effort, will gain the manifestation he deserves. This was known to the millions of lifestreams who first embodied on Earth. As will be presented later in this book, during the time period called the "Garden of Eden," all lifestreams did gain their ascension.

The Seven Bodies of Man

In order to embody upon the physical plane and go through the experience world, every individual must have seven bodies. Each body is created out of the substance of the realm in which it is to function.

The following is a brief description of the seven bodies.

ELECTRONIC BODY of the I AM PRESENCE. Its origin and function have already been described. It is the "real you," and it is anchored in the heart of your physical body. This creation is referred to in the Bible. "So God created man in his own image, in the image of God created he him." (Genesis 1:27) The electronic body of the I AM Presence is the God within us, and knows only perfection.

CAUSAL BODY of the I AM PRESENCE. The causal body, originally white, consists of seven concentric bands of color. The color of the first band is blue, and corresponds to the color of the first sphere. The colors of the other bands are identical to and correspond in sequence with the colors of the seven spheres. The first concentric band is the closest to the center. The causal body is always pictured as being around the electronic body of the I AM Presence. The head of the electronic body is the center of the causal body. The width of the bands signify how long the individual stayed within a particular sphere; the wider the band, the longer he stayed upon that sphere, thereby gaining additional development. The causal body contains the "Accumulated Good" — the opposite of Karma — which is the constructively qualified energy of the individual. (An illustration, published by A.D.K. Luk Publications shows the relationship between the Electronic Body of the I AM Presence, the causal body, the Christ Self and the physical body.)

THE CHRIST SELF (also called Holy Christ Self, or Higher Mental Body) abides in a position between the I AM Presence and the physical body. It is a replica (in form) of the I AM Presence, but vibrates at a lower rate. Operating at a lower vibration, it is aware of imperfection such as disease, but does not take it on and accept it.

The Christ Self may be considered the stepped-down transformer of the I AM Presence and it is ONE in action with it. It may also be considered the mediator between the individual's God-Self and his outer consciousness.

The Christ Self is the discriminative, directing intelligence through which the Presence works. It guides the personality, the outer self. It is "the still, small voice within," also called the guardian angel, sometimes giving promptings to do certain things. The number of promptings is usually three. If we do not follow these promptings, they will be discontinued after the third time.

THE ETHERIC BODY. In it are contained the memories of all past deeds, thoughts and feelings during former embodiments. The accumulation of these records is called the soul. The etheric body, therefore, is the envelope of the soul. (The definition of "soul" is based on a dictation by Lord Maitreya; other publications on this subject use a different meaning for "soul"). When an individual is not in embodiment, he lives in his etheric body, and has the consciousness of the soul.

The etheric body, as well as the emotional and mental bodies, interpenetrates the physical body. The shape of the etheric body is very similar to that of the physical body.

THE EMOTIONAL BODY, the largest of the four lower bodies, contains our feeling world. Its correct service is to nourish divine ideas with the positive feeling of accomplishment. It is oval in shape and extends at least three feet out from the physical body. Having total control of feelings is a desirable goal, often difficult to reach, especially for the occidental chela.

THE MENTAL BODY was designed to be the chalice for the receptivity of divine ideas. The mental body has the power to mold these ideas into workable form. The mind is contained in this body. The mind, also called consciousness, is to be the servant of the individualized flame, not its master. It was intended to be the instrument with which to create and hold the pattern or vision, until physical manifestation could take place.

THE PHYSICAL BODY provides the anchorage to the Earth. It is the vehicle through which man functions and expands the borders of God's kingdom into a lower vibratory plane. The physical body, therefore, is the temple of the living God.

Originally, this body was not as dense as it is now. It vibrated at a much higher level and it consisted of what we would today call etheric substance. Mankind, as it existed during the first Golden Age, would appear to us today as etheric, misty, shadowy beings, but of identical form as mankind today, if we could see these beings at all.

The silver cord enters the physical body at the top of the head (the soft spot of a newborn-baby), and provides the connection to the Christ-Self and the I AM Presence. It is the life-giving, life-maintaining fount of energy. If left without this fountain of life-force, the physical body could not operate, and so-called death would ensue.

The brain is the physical organ through which the mind functions. It registers impressions from the outer world. The brain is the vehicle of the mind.

The nervous system functions like a network of fine wires which are message bearers of thought and feeling impulses to all parts of the body. Through the spinal cord of every person two activities work constantly, the descending arc of electrical energy, which anchors the body on the surface of the Earth, and the powerful ascending current which enables one to stand erect and move about, rather than to crawl on the ground. When the activity of life is more powerfully charged into the ascending arc, we come to the point where the gravity pull of Earth no longer holds the lifestream, and ascension is possible.

The etheric, mental, and emotional bodies are not as intangible as one might think. Clairvoyants such as C.W. Leadbeater and Annie Besant were well aware of these bodies. They painted them, together with various thought forms, and published these pictures in the books, *Thoughtforms* and *Man Visible and Invisible*.

Also, it is possible that the effect of emotions can be seen through Kirlian photography. In one demonstration, the aura of the fingertip of an individual at peace with himself and the world showed up blue, whereas the same aura of a person in anger showed up as fire-engine red. In another test, a color photo done by high-energy photography showed predominantly gold colors. The individual, just before the photo was taken, had asked for divine guidance. I saw both of the original photos.

Guardian Spirits

Just before embodiment, each lifestream chosen by the Manu was brought before the Goddess of Liberty. Here he received the following encouraging message, "You are at liberty, beloved one, to take pure and primal life into the Earth plane. You are at liberty in the outer (the physical appearance) world to utilize life as you will. You are at liberty, beloved, to call upon any and all of Us (Ascended Beings) as you may choose, to assist you when the momentums and energy of your world seem not sufficient to handle the conditions necessary to fulfill your divine plan."

Then the call went forth for Guardian Spirits to assist those innocents, who were to find evolution upon the Earth. Guardian Spirits are lifestreams who have already gone through the same process of evolution upon another planet. They are older, more developed lifestreams. They may be ascended or unascended individuals. In gratitude for their service they are endowed by Helios with a jewel of light blazing from their foreheads.

In order to take voluntary embodiment on Earth, all lifestreams from other planets have to submit to the same laws, applicable to the Earth. The outer garments of the Guardian Spirits, therefore, are identical to those of the "innocents." They are of the same physical size and form.

Some Guardian Spirits took the vow never to ascend until all mankind is free. Many of these dear individuals are still with us today. The fact that they came originally from another planet is normally not known to any unascended being (the only one who can correctly tune into the Akashic Records of a former embodiment is an Ascended Master).

There came the time when the work of both creating the Earth and preparing the individualizations was complete, and the Earth was ready for habitation.

Purpose of Embodiment

Three distinct types of intelligent life were to be given opportunity to unfold their God-nature on our planet. These forms of life were angels, mankind, and elementals, each contributing in some manner to the well-being and progress of the other, and their combined life-force was ordained to weave the spiritual bridge to tie the Earth with the heart of God.

The purpose of embodiment is to master energy on a lower vibratory plane. Thus, in the denser substance of the Earth-plane, mankind learns how to wield the powers of thought, feeling, spoken word, action, and to consciously create as the Father does.

Creation is more difficult on a lower vibratory plane than on a higher one. Hence, individuals who have had this additional experience and have gained mastery have the opportunity to progress farther than those electing to have no embodiment.

Final Preparation of the Earth

Before the "Holy Innocents" were invited upon the Earth, Amaryllis, the Goddess of Spring, accompanied by legions of angelic and elemental helpers, clothed the Earth with the rhythm of spring in blossom, flower, and beauty of nature. The elementals wove the smallest and daintiest of flowers. The lotus was the first flower brought forth on Earth. Nature Devas unfolded the leaves of the trees. To the tune of the rhythmic music of creation, nature worked together for 900 springs in this process of beautification to adorn the Earth for the descent of man. There were the rivers, the waterfalls, the mountains, the lakes, the oceans, the trees, the other lush vegetation. With its alabaster-like surface the Earth sparkled like a jewel; it was a beautiful thing to behold.

2 - The First Two Golden Ages - The Garden Of Eden

MAN'S ADVENT ON EARTH

After Amaryllis, the Goddess of Spring, completed her task, the Seven-Fold Flame of the Elohim signified to the world that the Earth was ready for habitation.

It was the twenty-first of March, and the beginning of the spring solstice, when Helios and Vesta chose to bring down for embodiment the first subrace of the first rootrace. The year was not stated in equally precise terms; however, from the data given by the Masters, this event probably occurred about 4-1/2 million years ago. (Further discussion on this subject will be found under the chapter "The Age of Man.")

Present besides the members of the first rootrace were Helios and Vesta, members of the angelic kingdom, including Archangel Michael, the directors of the earth, water, and air elements, namely Virgo,

Neptune and Aries, the Maha Chohan, the Manu of the first rootrace and guardian spirits. Among the Guardian Spirits present were Sanat Kumara, an Ascended Being from Venus, and Zarathustra, a being from the Central Sun, representing the fire-element.

A gigantic light ray was projected from the sun, and the majestic descent to the Earth began. Archangel Michael was the first to touch the surface of the Earth. He vowed that he would give assistance to all mankind, until the last lifestream gained his ascension. Then the Maha Chohan established the Flame of the Holy Spirit and the Comfort Flame.

The descent occurred in the vicinity of the Teton Mountains (Wyoming). This Rocky Mountain Retreat is the most ancient focus of the Ascended Masters upon the Earth. It is also called the Temple of Precipitation. Precipitation means "going forth," and this refers to man's advent on Earth. From here the newborn men went North, East, South and West to carry the Light of God to the four corners of the Earth.

THE GARDEN OF EDEN

Man in the Garden Of Eden

"And God saw everything that he had made and behold, it was very good." (Genesis 1:31) This account refers to the first two Golden Ages and the first three rootraces, during which time there was no imperfection. Mankind lived in the Garden of Eden, E-Don meaning obedience to divine wisdom, the all-knowing activity of consciousness. During this time period no lifestream used energy to create a discordant vibration. The Earth was as harmonious as heaven. Each individual was part of a great symphony, and in complete obedience to his Christ Self and his I AM Presence. Each one's inner bodies were vibrating in perfect harmony. Mankind's attention rested upon the things above, not upon things of the Earth.

We may ask, "What was man's appearance at this time?" Since the vibrations of his garments were much higher than those of today, man's physical body at this time was of lesser density, and could be compared to the present etheric body, which is of vapor-like substance. Therefore, it is unlikely that the members of the first three rootraces left any fossil evidence.

During this Golden Age man's bodies were luminous. As far as his hands could reach there was a self-luminous radiance, visible to the outer sight of everyone. No deception was possible because the color of the radiance showed thought and feeling. Mankind looked as our Christ-Self looks today. Since the luminosity of the electrons shone through the outer garment, no artificial lighting was required. Day and night as we experience them today were unknown.

The blazing sphere of pure white light formed a natural armour of protection, keeping out rates of vibration that did not belong to the perfection of the Presence. (Students of Ascended Master Teaching know how to re-establish this protective armour of light today.)

This was a period of time when everyone could see his own I AM Presence, and walked and talked with the angels and Ascended Beings. There was no veil between them.

Through the power of thought and feeling, men designed and precipitated the requirement of the moment, whether it was food, clothing, shelter, or lovely temples. Through the power of feeling man energized thought forms by using universal light-substance. All that was drawn forth was used for the good of the whole. Every man, woman and child was about the Father's business. All were interested only in widening the borders of the kingdom, by coalescing into form the divine ideas which daily passed from the I AM Presence of each individual into his outer consciousness through the silver cord. Each lifestream was like a fountain, drawing forth new ideas from the Presence, coalescing around himself elemental substance, which responded instantly to his call, since he was a co-creator with God.

So many magnificent ideas poured forth in one day that the outer self could not fulfill them all. The outer self then chose those ideas which would be of the greatest blessing to the universe.

Whatever man did in those early ages, he did well and in great detail. Many hours, months, or even a lifetime was often spent in carving out one figure or weaving one rug.

Those were days of great happiness and beauty, and there existed only perfection in every avenue of life. The "curse of Cain" (labor by the sweat of the brow), disintegration, and death were unknown.

Religious Life

Education, science, and religion were not thought of as separate subjects. There was only one subject, namely, God and His ideas. The Glory of the One was manifested in all walks of life.

Certain lifestreams, utilizing their individuality, became specialists and entered the priesthood. They were trained in temples to become experts in precipitation, education and healing. Whenever mankind felt depleted in one quality or another, they visited these temples and were revitalized.

The Temple of Illumined Faith was located near Banff, British Columbia. It was originally carved out of a mountain. Lord Michael served here, and his wise counsel was lovingly obeyed. People came individually and in groups to absorb the consciousness of absolute faith in God's goodness.

The Freedom Flame was kept at the Freedom Temple, and served to accelerate the externalization of the individual's divine plan, thereby hastening his development. The Freedom Flame, (purple in color), is an activity of the Seventh Ray. During this time the amethyst was permitted to be worn only by the priests of the Order of Archangel Zadkiel.

Pallas Athena, Goddess of Truth, was High Priestess at the Temple of Truth. The pilgrims would visit her to gain from the magnetizing effect of the green Flame of Truth.

Other guardian spirits, among them The Great Divine Director, Lanto, Surya, and Kwan Yin, together with the angelic host, walked and talked with the members of the first three rootraces on a daily basis.

The seven Archangels held the offices of the seven Chohans. Chohan means "lord of the ray." Each Chohan was, and to this day is, responsible for one ray. The Maha Chohan (great lord of rays) was, and is, in charge of the seven Chohans.

Archangel Jophiel was the First World Teacher. Among others who later represented this office were Gautama Buddha, Lord Maitreya, and Jesus.

Individual Re-embodiment

During the first two Golden Ages, the physical bodies for new Earth inhabitants were created by the parents by means of light rays. Through the projection of two rays, (one of a masculine and one of a feminine being), a new body was created at the point where the rays crossed. This body was formed to full stature; infancy was unknown. Then the incoming lifestream took possession of the newly-created form. Each individual life-span lasted for thousands of years, since the vibration of each electron, atom, and cell was held in harmony with the Presence.

Toward the end of an embodiment the individual informed his relatives and friends of his coming transition. Then he searched for new parents, and, having their consent, left with them some of his earthly possessions, such as books and research papers.

Now the individual stepped into the Transmuting Violet Flame, which was anchored and maintained by the priesthood in a temple. The flame instantly etherealized the physical form, and the elements returned to be universal life substance. The lifestream's memory record, also called the soul, entered inner realms for a time and was drawn back later at a self-chosen time by the individual. This way he obtained the full memory of his past life or lives. He was then ready for another embodiment, and for renewed opportunity for growth and fulfillment of his divine plan.

"A minimum of seven embodiments, one for each ray, was necessary to gain the ascension. This process occurred without interruption during the first two Golden Ages, whereby the first three rootraces flourished, and all members of these rootraces gained their ascension."

Climate and Surroundings

During the first two Golden Ages mankind enjoyed a semi-tropical, even climate. There were no storms and adverse weather conditions to combat. Also, there was perfect harmony and rhythm in the change of the seasons. The four seasons served to give variation in color and design, as well as variations in types of harvest.

Lush foliage covered the ground; there were no weeds, bugs, insects, vermin, or diseases. Also, no volcanoes were present. All volcanic action is due to the antipathy between elementals and mankind, whom they had come in such love to serve.

Animals, as we know them today, were not yet in existence. They only began to appear after humanity had generated the discord that followed the first two Golden Ages. Birds, however, fall under a separate category. They were created by Ascended Beings as messengers to mankind. Some did later take on some human qualities, which accounts for their destructive activities.

In the first two Golden Ages the landed surfaces were connected all around the Earth. There were oceans as well. No icecaps were present. The latter were caused by mankind's coldness and bitterness, and they will disappear when mankind radiates more love. The name of one of the continents in existence at that time was Lemuria, also called Mu.

The surface of the Earth was white, like alabaster or white quartz, radiating iridescent colors of the rainbow. There were rivers, waterfalls, lakes, oceans, trees and other vegetation, and mountains. "Highly developed Beings, called Gods of the Mountains, have sustained those mountains against the gravity pull of the Earth through love, from the beginning of time. They have held them like great spires pointing heavenward, directing mankind's attention toward God."

The First Four Rootraces

The first subrace of the first rootrace came to North America. It embodied first in the vicinity of the Tetons. No information was given as to where the second rootrace was located.

The third rootrace and forerunners of the fourth rootrace came in in the vicinity of the Fiji Islands, then part of the gigantic continent of Lemuria. The entire third rootrace flourished on Lemuria, while the remainder of the fourth rootrace embodied in Eastern Asia and upon Atlantis.

Lemuria was a large land mass covering parts of the Pacific Ocean. Its eastern coast reached to the area around San Diego, California. Australia, New Zealand, Hawaii, and the Fiji Islands were part of Lemuria.

The Masters explained that there has never been a land so fair outside the kingdom of heaven, where man walked in such grace and beauty, as in China during its Golden Age. It was impossible to distinguish the Ascended Beings from the evolving ones on Earth.

During the Golden Age of China, Kwan Yin, the Goddess of Mercy, together with the twelve ladies of her spiritual court, walked and talked with the people of her country. She was an unascended master at that time, and gave audiences in the larger cities of China, as well as in her retreat in Peking.

In those days, beauty and harmony were the keynote

of China, and an entire embodiment was spent in the carving of one miniature, the painting of a single flower, or the weaving of one lovely robe of state. Messengers were sent from all over the world to invite the scholars, the priests, and the teachers of China to bring their culture to the youth of all lands. Everyone in that empire was as consciously aware of the I AM Presence as the man of today is aware of his hands and feet.

Kwan Yin ministered for over 1,000 years to the people of Eastern Asia before accepting the freedom of her ascension.

3 - The Fall Of Man

THE LAGGARDS

It was during the incoming of the fourth rootrace, that a Cosmic Council convened whose decision changed drastically the course for all evolutions of Earth's mankind, guardian spirits, angels and elementals.

This Council, attended by the spiritual Hierarchy of the Earth, was called to decide what to do with billions of lifestreams who lived in another galaxy. These lifestreams were of insufficient spiritual development to earn continued habitation upon their own planet for evolution. As part of the divine plan, their planet was to undergo one step of the inbreath, bringing it one step closer to the sun.

According to Cosmic Law, closer proximity to the sun requires an acceleration of the vibration of a planet and its inhabitants. The individuals refused to go along with the divine plan. They were complacent in their thoughts and feelings, and lagged behind in their natural process of evolution. Hence they were not qualified to move forward with their planet. Those individuals were referred to by the Masters as "laggards."

One plan was to have them pass through what we call "second death," which ends the life of the individual by reducing his components to universal substance, from which there is no coming back. It was then that the Hierarchy of Earth, as an act of mercy, offered the Earth as a planetary home to help the laggards complete their evolution. Conditions on this planet were still perfect and harmonious, yet compared to other planets, its vibratory rate was slightly slower. It was hoped that the laggards would be guided by the purity and perfection of the thoughts and feelings of the people of the Earth, and by holding to this example, they would gradually transmute their karma. The High Priests and Guardian Spirits were informed of the coming of the laggards; the remainder of mankind was unaware of the event. For one hundred years the High Priests attempted, through decreeing, to establish a shield around the Earth's lifestreams to prevent their contamination by the laggards.

What did the laggards look like after they came to Earth? Tied now to the same laws which applied to the remainder of mankind on Earth, they were provided with similar bodies, and therefore were not distinguishable from the rest.

The chief faults of the laggards were arrogance, rebellion, resistance to progress, stubbornness and resentment toward change. Naturally, they brought these qualities with them. The impure thoughtforms of the laggards spread into Earth's atmosphere like smog. It was the beginning of the "mist" the Bible talks about ("and a mist arose and covered the whole ground," Gen. 2:6).

In time the people of Earth succumbed to the subtle

temptation of curiosity. They tuned in to the impure thought-forms of the laggards, and started to play with them. This experimentation with the misuse of free will caused what is known as the "fall of man." Mankind started to listen to the "wrong crowd." Independent of God-direction, mankind deliberately chose to experiment with impurity. This way man's attention no longer rested exclusively on his inner Presence, the director of his life-activity. Man became sense-conscious, instead of God-conscious, and so, according to Cosmic Law, manifested that upon which his attention was directed and which he thought about most. He deliberately and consciously turned his back upon the perfection and dominion with which the Father endowed him from the beginning.

When the mist first appeared, it was like a local wisp of smoke. Later, as the ages passed, it became an increasing fog, that gradually shut away the visible presence of the Ascended Host.

Thus, the glory of perfection of the first two Golden Ages came to an end. Later on, when the Atlantean culture flourished, there were other Golden Ages, during which the veil between the Ascended Host and mankind was partially rent; however, the perfection of the first two Golden Ages was unique and was never quite matched. The Masters assured the students that it is possible for us to rent the veil again, and that man once more may be able to walk and talk with the Ascended Host and the angels.

The laggards did not come to Earth all at once. All together there were billions of them.

DISHARMONY APPEARS

The Masters stated that the "fall of man" occurred on today's Australia and New Zealand. At that time these countries were part of the gigantic continent of Mu, which covered a large part of the Pacific and Indian Oceans. It was here that slander and gossip first began the weave of the veil.

In order to assign a time for the "fall of man" we may reason that the Ascended Masters stated repeatedly that there were two Golden Ages during which there was no imperfection. Also, based on the previous discussion of "Rootraces and Cycles," we know that under perfect conditions it takes a cycle of 14,000 years for one rootrace to make the ascension. Furthermore, it was made clear that the first three rootraces experienced no imperfection and gained their ascension during the appointed time. In addition, we know that the laggards arrived at the beginning of the incoming of the fourth rootrace, indirectly causing the end of a state of absolute perfection on Earth. Therefore, if we chose to define the "fall of man" as the time when disharmony first appeared on Earth, we may assign a date of about 50,000 years after mankind first appeared upon this globe.

The above account appears to conflict with a dictation by the Ascended Master Krishna. He stated that when the "fall" occurred and the mist covered the whole ground, one million years had passed (measured from the time man first appeared upon Earth). However, there is not necessarily a conflict. As pointed out previously, it took ages until the mist, originally just a local wisp of smoke, became an increasing fog that gradually shut away the visible presence of the Ascended Host. Therefore, it depends upon one's definition of the "fall." If one chooses to define it as the time when disharmony first appeared, on the basis on unerring Cosmic Law, we can assign a time period of 50,000 years. If we choose to define the "fall" as the time when a mist covered ALL of the ground surface of the Earth, we can assign a time period of one million years.

CONSEQUENCES OF THE FALL

Effect on Priesthood

After the arrival of the laggards, the priesthood split into two factions. Rather than listening to the plan devised by the Hierarchy, one section of the priesthood attempted to remove the laggards away from the Earth through repeated invocations. One Ascended Master explained the senselessness of this operation. Even if the attempt would have succeeded, the laggards, bound to the laws of the Earth just as the original races were, would have had to come before the Karmic Board and would have necessarily had to re-enter the Earth. Therefore, no permanent removal would have been possible. The dictations seem to suggest that the other faction of the priesthood accepted the laggards, refusing to rebel against the plan of the Hierarchy.

Effect on Individual Man

The "fall of man" into a lower vibratory level caused great changes in mankind's bodily structure.

The form grew more dense, and creation by light-rays came to an end. Also, the I AM Presence, the focus of light and life in the heart center, began to decrease in size and influence. Fear, for the first time, registered in the etheric body, and the soul was born. The soul may be called the accumulated records from the experimental use of life. This soul, dwelling in the etheric body, later influenced each personality in each succeeding embodiment. The soul has to be redeemed through constructively-qualified energy until there are no longer two — the soul and divine consciousness — but rather, God alone. Re-acquiring this God consciousness is the need of the hour. It is "the second coming of the Christ."

The growing density of the physical body caused changes in man's bodily form, and for the first time man experienced the present form of birth.

The veil, once it was in total effect, shut off the visible presence of Divine Beings; also, the Music of the Spheres could no longer be heard. The outer consciousness was left in confusion, groping in darkness.

Commencing with the "fall," very few individuals gained their ascension. Nearly everybody, through the misuse of energy, acquired karma, and this way became tied to the wheel of birth and rebirth.

Effect on Guardian Spirits

After the "fall of man," some of the Guardian Spirits remained in bodies of Light, choosing not to take on the newly-created bodies of man. Among them were Kwan Yin and the Great Divine Director. They asked for, and were granted their ascension.

However, some of the guardians chose to enter the

new garments of flesh, hoping to thereby hold a connection with the ascended Guardian Spirits through the veil. Thus occurred the first parting of these unselfish individuals, with only intuition and the feeling of the heart giving a clue to the former connection.

As the centuries passed, the unascended guardian spirits also became enmeshed in their karma, forgetting their origin and source, thereby tying themselves to the wheel of birth and rebirth. Kwan Yin stated to the students that it was the great sacrifice of the Guardian Spirits that has warranted the special attention for the Earth by the Ascended Masters, and also has justified the endless patience for the remainder of mankind.

Effect on Hierarchy of the Earth

Before the "fall" there existed only a Liberating Council, consisting of three members. There was no discord, therefore there was no need for judgement.

After the "fall," the Liberating Council was replaced by the Karmic Board, consisting of seven members, one for each ray. It is the purpose of the Karmic Board to place the incoming lifestreams in such a position as to make possible redemption for wrongdoing.

Effect on the Surface of the Earth

Before the "fall" the pigment of the Earth's surface was an alabaster color. After the "fall" the pigment started changing, and the grays and browns appeared. It took a long time before black and red appeared (here we are talking about fire-engine red); it was not until 80,000 years ago that these colors manifested.

After the fall, the centripetal force, creating the law of gravity, which holds the landed surface and people on the Earth, had to be adjusted from time to time, in proportion to the density of the physical bodies of mankind. (Centripetal force in curvilinear motion is the force which tends to pull an object rotating around a center, towards that center; it is the opposite of centrifugal force.)

The discord of mankind created, in some instances, so much disharmony that the nature kingdom refused to continue doing its part in adorning the Earth with foliage. As a result, the first barren wastelands and deserts appeared. Some of today's soil-conservationists and environmentalists are persons, who through the mercy of the Karmic Board, are placed in those positions so they can make restitution for their past misdeeds.

Man's misqualified energy brought about gas-belts, subterranean pressure chambers, which, under certain conditions, result in earthquakes and volcanic action. (The location of these gas-belts is described in James Churchward's *The Second Book of the Cosmic Forces of Mu.*) Later on the gas belts were responsible for the sinking of that portion of Mu located where the Pacific Ocean now is.

ANIMALS

During the first two Golden Ages there were no animals as we know them today, and no vicious creations. All elemental forms were beautiful, and individually outpictured God's perfection. The angelic, devic (nature) and elemental kingdoms had preceded mankind in order to prepare a place for them. The elementals were destined to accompany man, to serve him, and to be obedient to him throughout his pilgrimage on Earth.

The repellent octopus of today was once a lovely, golden miniature sun. Instead of tentacles there were rays of iridescent light, that poured forth in the water element. The oyster and clam of today were once beautiful little fairy forms.

The oyster and clam created a shell, and the rhinoceros, the buffalo, and elephant, once beautiful, developed thick, coarse skin or hair as a protection, as a defense mechanism against the vicious currents in the earth's atmosphere. Horns, hooves and scales come under the same category. The dinosaur age was the darkest point in the Earth's history. The prehistoric mammal and the ape were vicious creations caused by man's misuse of energy.

Animals have ganglionic centers and emotional bodies; plant life does not. It is life energy that beats the heart of the animals, not an individualized Flame of God as in the case of mankind. Within the heart of these imprisoned elementals is the pattern which they once displayed and which pattern they are to outpicture again.

The effects upon the nature kingdom were similar. Plant life developed weeds, thorns, poison, and heavy bark.

There is but one road to freedom for all life, and that is through love. Love is the primal essence, and the development of this quality in the individual consciousness is the only means by which any expressions of life can be set free.

Great men and women, such as Ascended Master Kuthumi in his embodiment as Saint Francis of Assisi, have loved hundreds of thousands of animals free. Through love and association their consciousness was raised to the point where they did not have to come back into animal form. Some lifestreams volunteer, before coming into a particular embodiment, to assist the elemental kingdom. In this way they can transmute some wrongdoing from a previous embodiment.

Whether or not a person should have a pet living with him in his home is his own personal decision. Any close proximity to an animal — as is the case also with another person — may have a possible adverse effect on the aura (the surrounding energy field of the individual, similar in shape to the physical body, but slightly larger). It should, however, also be considered, that the student has the capability through the strength of its own sphere of influence to be the "leaven in the loaf" of the lesser intelligence. Balance should be the key in today's relationship with animals. There is no reason to be extreme in one's sentiment regarding these creatures. A steady middle course is required, enfolding in thought and feeling all expressions on this Earth in tolerance, patience, and love, thereby raising this innocent life into its former state of freedom and perfection.

THE FIRST WORLD SAVIOUR

During the first two Golden Ages there was absolute perfection. There was the activity of teaching and learning, but nobody needed assistance "to be saved."

The first Christ was provided for mankind when man first chose to become sense-conscious instead of remaining God-conscious. Man directed his attention toward the pains and pleasures of the five senses, and thereby manifested that to which his attention was directed and upon which he thought most.

Since that time, 49 World Saviours have come to Earth at regular intervals. The First Christ was Krishna. He drew to Earth the Resurrection Flame, as a means of restoring the fallen sons of God, in case they desired to return to their natural God-Estate. This flame was necessary for mankind, for the nature kingdom and for elemental life to rebuild an imperfect form created by imperfect thought and feelings. The Resurrection Flame contains the resurrecting power, without which man cannot enter into his Christ-Estate.

Krishna came from the Central Sun. It was not possible to draw upon the lifestreams of the Earth at that time, because they were still children in their spiritual development, and because nearly all of them "had already eaten from the forbidden fruit." From the small group that had maintained a pure consciousness, other Christs, such as Buddha and Jesus, would later be developed.

There were several Krishnas. The first Krishna stayed upon the Earth for several hundred years. He taught his disciples that "Service is the Law of Life." Krishna explained that an individual should accept the responsibility for giving a balance to the universe for the privilege of drawing breath, using life, and sustaining a separate, individual existence.

Krishna emphasized that service should be impersonal, for love's sake, and without any thought of remuneration. As an example of impersonal service Krishna pointed to the sun. He stated, "Peace comes only, when to the best of your ability, you are endeavoring to serve the cause of good and have no concern for any external activity, in relation to its effects upon your service."

Service may be in the form of serving a community,

a nation, or a fellow man. Individuals who do not choose to serve are temporarily taken out of the race until they will accept again their responsibility to be conscious servants.

Some of Krishna's instructions were preserved by his disciples by inscribing them on rolls of linen, which were coated with a soft wax. The linen then was rolled on spindles of bamboo, the entire document sometimes covering several hundred feet. Through these documents, he left a heritage upon which all of the Vedas and other most ancient writings are based. These documents survived cataclysm after cataclysm, and were moved by the wise and elect across the face of the earth.

Krishna abided upon the Earth for at least 640 years. When He completed his service and returned to His star, He took with him 1,400 disciples, who through His service, gained their ascension.

4 - The Age Of Man

INTRODUCTION

The question, "When did man first set foot on this globe?" has puzzled many throughout the ages. Depending upon the source, the answer varies from 4004 B.C. to millions of years.

Bishop James Ussher, using the Bible as a reference, arrived at the date 4004 B.C. Most archaeologists, geologists, and other natural scientists believe man evolved over a period of millions of years.

We can consider ourselves fortunate, indeed, that the Ascended Masters — after the occult law was set aside in 1930 — were able to give us certain dates, enabling us to answer the question at hand with some certainty. No longer do we have to ponder about the veiled occult data of the East. This is the information Helen Blavatsky desired, but which could not be given by the Masters under occult law, which prevailed during her time.

THE DATA EXAMINED

The instructions given by various Ascended Masters through the two messengers concerning the age of man may be separated into the following categories:

1) The time period covering man's existance on Earth.
2) The time period before the "veil" shut down the visible presence of the Ascended Host.
3) The time period thereafter, when mankind "lived in the shadows."

An analysis of the time periods above enables us to check the information as to the total age of man.

Data Relating to Total Age of Mankind

When researching this item, I found the following references:

"All should understand that human beings have lived upon the Earth for more than 4 million years." (Elohim Vista, also called Cyclopea)

"That Light which is your accumulation of good for 4-1/2 million years..." (Archangel Michael) (He was talking about the accumulation of good in each embodiment, which is stored in the causal body.)

"The words 'I AM' are the mightiest words in any language that has come forth for the use of mankind in 4-1/2 million years. They are the signal to all forces of light to come into action at your point in the universe." (Archangel Michael)

"The words 'I AM,' as written in English today, have come down from the beginning of mankind's appearance on Earth. In the Grand Teton (Retreat) there are records of these civilizations, every one which has ever been on Earth; and every one of these civilizations used the words 'I AM' as written in English today, showing that these two words are the word of God." (Great Divine Director)

"In every civilization that has ever been on Earth the words 'I AM' have been used as written in English today." (Cuzco)

Sanat Kumara was one of the original guardian spirits who came 4-1/2 million years ago from Venus to assist the Earth. 2-1/2 million years ago, when the Earth's accumulated, constructive energy was at its low point, and man had degraded to the point where he became a caveman, Sanat Kumara volunteered to contribute His own accumulated energy to the Earth as a balance, taking residence at Shamballa, thereby saving the Earth from dissolution. (See next chapter.) This action was different from being a guardian spirit.

"Sanat Kumara has guarded the Earth for these 4-1/2 million years." (Jesus)

"Sanat Kumara for 4-1/2 million years has blessed the Earth with His presence." (Cosmic Being Victory)

"Venus, of its own volition, chose to assist the Earth and has, for 4-1/2 million years." (Goddess of Peace)

"My great teacher, Sanat Kumara, for 4-1/2 million years has watched over the Earth." (Cosmic Being Victory)

"I came forth from Venus by my own volition, 4-1/2 million years ago, to assist the people on Earth." (Sanat Kumara)

"Through the Kumaras as the vanguard from Venus, mankind has been sustained for more than 4 million years." (Mr. Rayborn, an Ascended Being)

"Guardian Spirits came from Venus, Uranus, Mercury, and other stars. Some, such as Sanat Kumara, were already ascended." (Kwan Yin)

"I reigned in America when there was absolute perfection. That seed was planted more than 3 million years ago." (Archangel Michael)

Data Relating to Man's Perfection

The time period covering the length of the Garden of Eden, when man lived in a state of absolute perfection, was previously established at 50,000 years, and the time when the "veil" totally covered the surface of the Earth, was probably one million years after man first set foot on the globe. The Master Krishna chose to label this event as the "Fall of Man." (See chapter "Fall of Man," Section "Disharmony Appears.")

The following is a statement of Cosmic Being Victory, "For two million years mankind lived in a state of magnificent perfection."

This statement does not necessarily suggest a conflict with the preceding data. The question here seems to be, is "absolute perfection" equal to "magnificent perfection?" There seems to be no doubt what "absolute perfection" means. It means the time during which mankind lived in the Garden of Eden and there was no disharmony.

"Magnificent perfection," however, appears to refer to a level of perfection, and depends on the point of reference of the beholder. What does he compare it to? For example, if we compare the state of perfection of the Sahara Civilization with today's conditions, we could rightfully say the Sahara Civilization achieved a state of magnificent perfection. If, however, we compare the same civilization with the conditions of the first two Golden Ages, the Garden of Eden, we could not use the term "magnificent perfection." Similarly, when compared to today's conditions, perhaps the one-million or two-million-year-period after the advent of man may be termed "magnificent perfection."

The Time When Man "Lived in the Shadows"

"For two and a half million years mankind misused life, played with it, and wrongly qualified it. Now the Great Cosmic Light has said, 'No longer may you misuse and wrongly qualify life, since you have now become intelligent beings.'" (Cosmic Being Victory)

"You have lived in mistakes for two and a half million years." (Cosmic Being Victory)

"Here we are operating within the Earth's sphere, dissolving, consuming, and forever removing the viciousness of those who are inhabitants of the psychic or astral plane, which is the destructive force generated and created by mankind through two-and-one-half million years." (Goddess of Light)

"You (the students of the Light) are rendering a service to the Earth which I have required for more than two million years." (Sanat Kumara) He took up residence in Shamballa and became Lord of the World, two and a half million years ago.

"Never has there been, in the history of the Earth, for two and a half million years, such magnificent, practical understanding as you have within your hands today." (Great Divine Director)

"After two and a half million years, many times in various parts of the Earth, humanity did reach a very high state, but no civilization, no people can ever have a permanently-sustained attainment until they have known the I AM Presence which gives life to Earth. Those civilizations did not know what you are privileged to know today." (Sanat Kumara)

"The decrees have rendered a service to the world like nothing in two million years has done." (Sanat Kumara)

"Since mankind has had more than three million years to go through birth and rebirth, those of today who have the opportunity and privilege of gaining the ascension should not contemplate sex." (Goddess of Purity)

SUMMARY

The data indicates that man first appeared upon this globe about four million years ago, on the twenty-first of March, during the spring solstice. This historic event occurred in the neighborhood of the Teton Mountains and is further described under the chapter "Advent of Man."

Broadly speaking, we may divide mankind's development into three major stages:

1) The Garden of Eden
After mankind came to Earth there were 50,000 years of absolute perfection, ending when the first laggard came and disharmony first appeared.

2) 50,000 years after man's advent on Earth, to about 3 million years ago
This time period lasted probably one million years, and was characterized by man gradually forgetting his source and reaching a lower state of accomplishment. In the beginning of this time period

there were just "localized puffs of smoke" in the atmosphere. At the end of this period there was a total veil, shutting off the visible presence of the Ascended Host.

3) Three million years ago to the present

This period was called by the Masters, "mankind living in the shadows." Within this span, the low point of our civilization was reached about two and a half million years ago.

5 - Sanat Kumara Saves The Earth

THE LOW POINT IN OUR HISTORY

Once the laggards were brought to Earth, mankind started its downward trend. The "local mist" (Genesis 2:6) caused by the laggards became a total veil, generated when most of mankind tuned into thoughtforms of misqualified energy and produced some of their own. This downward trend continued until the Earth reached such a low point that it became a concern of the Hierarchy of its galaxy.

Cosmic Law demands any planet to carry a certain amount of Light (harmoniously, constructively-qualified energy) by its inhabitants as a condition of maintaining its place in a solar system. About two and a half million years ago, during the Mu-Age (Lemurian Age), the Earth fell short on the following counts:

1) It did not emit sufficient constructive radiation.

2) It did not contribute sufficiently to the music of the galaxy, the so-called "Music of the Spheres."

3) Its rotating axis was tilted 45 degrees. If this would have gone farther, it would have been disastrous. [Now, in 1983, it is tilted about 23 degrees.]

4) Guardian spirits cannot stay indefinitely on a planet. They must return to their own planets, their natural sphere of activity. Their place must be taken by the natural lifestreams of the Earth. This

has not occurred. THE FIRST THREE ROOTRACES ASCENDED, BUT OUT OF THESE MILLIONS OR BILLIONS OF LIFESTREAMS, NOT A SINGLE INDIVIDUAL CONTRIBUTED IN ANY MANNER TO THE SUCCEEDING RACES. All of these individuals chose to progress at inner levels, and thereby elected not to assist the inhabitants of the Earth.

5) Man descended to the stage known to us as the caveman. Even the knowledge of how to make a simple fire became a forgotten item. The age of the dinosaurs prevailed.

6) The spark in the heart of the individual, which maintains his life, and which anchors the I AM Presence, had shrunk to one sixteenth of an inch.

7) The nature kingdom revolted and refused to bring forth any new foliage for a mankind so full of discord and lack of appreciation of their services.

Against the backdrop of these alarming developments, Helios and Vesta were required to attend a Cosmic Council. The Council was attended by representatives of the galaxy of which the Earth is part, as well as by representatives from other galaxies. The conference was chaired by Alpha and Omega, who are responsible for our galaxy.

After considering all pertinent factors, a proposal was made to write off the Earth as a useless experience. As part of this plan, the Earth was to be swung off its axis, thereby dissolving it. This would have meant "SECOND DEATH" for its inhabitants, from which there is no coming back into embodiment, and therefore complete annihilation forever of all life on Earth.

Sanat Kumara, an Ascended Being from the planet Venus, and one of its regents, at this point suggested that if an Ascended Being with sufficient Light (constructively-qualified energy) chose to remain in the Earth-atmosphere and offer His Light as a balance for the Light-quota lacking on Earth, the

Earth might be saved. This would have to be done until some of the lifestreams belonging to the Earth (not including guardian spirits) could be trained to take His place.

Archangel Raphael agreed, and asked for volunteers. Sanat Kumara indicated he would be interested provided that his twin-flame, Venus, the other Co-Regent of the planet Venus, would consent. Venus subsequently agreed, and this freed Sanat Kumara to proceed with His mission.

It was stated to the students in the 1950's that Sanat Kumara had fulfilled similar missions before, each time returning home victorious. [From this account it is reasonable to assume that a similar "Fall of Man" also took place on other planets.] In the Bible Sanat Kumara is called "the Ancient of Days" (Daniel 7:9).

PREPARATION FOR SHAMBALLA

After returning to his home-star Venus, Sanat Kumara made the announcement of his offer to His people. Inspired by His example of selfless love, 30 priests [in other dictations this number was given as 100] from the planet Venus offered to precede him to prepare a place for him. They imprinted into their memory the City of Shamballa on Venus, which was to serve as a model for Sanat Kumara's home on Earth. Then they bade goodbye to their families, their home, and their planet, and stood before the Lords of Karma of the Earth. This great Council accepted the offer of the volunteers with great gratitude.

There were no special privileges accorded to these priests. They were bound to the laws of the Earth, including the wheel of re-embodiment, and each one was to understand that he had to share Sanat Kumara's destiny, namely, none would be released until the hour came when the Earth's own Light was sufficient to meet the demand of Cosmic Law. They were not granted the privilege of consecutive consciousness, and had to submit to the "Bands of Forgetfulness," an act of mercy which applies to all unascended lifestreams of the Earth. Were it not for this act of mercy, mankind would be troubled with the memory of thousands of embodiments, which according to the Masters, would give us too much to handle at one time. Therefore, all that was left of the memory of Venus was the imprint on their etheric bodies of the picture of Shamballa as it existed on Venus, or the promptings of their hearts. There was to be no Master showing them the way on Earth, and no other outer assistance given.

When the priests awoke in infant form they looked the same as any other individual on Earth at that time. They were born in different countries; some were born in North America.

After they reached adulthood, the former priests of Venus followed their heart's promptings, causing some to leave their families. A part of those living in the area today called the United States gathered near what is now New York City. They had one thing in common, an inner memory of a shining city. They crossed several great seas and continents. Some of the former priests finally gathered on the mainland, close to the Gobi Sea, a large body of water which is now the Gobi Desert. Many had had a wearisome journey, but a burning desire lighted their way, and let them remember their purpose sufficiently to find their pilgrim brothers. After arriving upon the shores of the Gobi Sea, the strongest among them brought forth a vision of their purpose, and it was confirmed in the hearts of the others. Thus started the preparation of what is known as "the building of Shamballa."

THE EARTH, 2.5 MILLION YEARS AGO

Let us pause here a moment to reflect upon some of the details which the Masters gave us on the topography of the Earth at that time.

According to one dictation, the present Gobi Desert was a large inland sea, and its sapphire-blue waters dashed against the Himalayan Mountains. Another dictation speaks of "swiftly moving waters." This suggests that the large body of water called the "Gobi Sea" had at least one inlet and one outlet. "There were hills not too far from the Gobi Sea, occupied by savage members of the human race. They were the Laggards." [There is evidence that at one time there was indeed a Gobi Sea. A geologist, Professor Rehwinkel, stated that the territory now known as the Gobi Desert was at one time a large inland lake as large as the Mediterranean Sea. "The existence of this inland sea is attested to by the abundant sedimentary deposit around the circumference and also by the Chinese historical reference to it as the 'Great Han Hai,' or the Great Interior Sea."]

The dictation which told of the priests starting out from the United States mentioned they had to cross several great seas and continents, and several other dictations suggest that from the beginning of time there were always several continents above water. Cosmic Law tends to support this view. The overcrowding of this planet caused by allowing billions of laggards to occupy it, makes it mandatory for the Karmic Lords to continually find new opportunities for unascended lifestreams to redeem their karma. Therefore, large amounts of land have to be above water on a continual basis.

THE BUILDING OF SHAMBALLA

Within the Gobi Sea there was an island with lush green foliage, upon which it was decided to build Shamballa. This island was later called "White Island."

Drawn together by the bonds of common interest in one cause, the next task of the 30 volunteers was to find the material of which Shamballa was to be built, and by the labor of their own hands, design and build from marble and stone the vision which they held within their minds. Conditions were similar to those encountered today. There was no special assistance given these individuals. There was a veil, and there was no coming and going of visible angelic beings.

"From all over the world they carried by the sweat of the brow and not in mystic chariot, all the tremendous pieces of marble and the various other heavy stones that formed the mighty edifices. They used the most beautiful materials the Earth could offer. Some among them, who were powerful in the use of magnetization, helped them in the erecting of some of these stones, weighing tons."

The latter statement may be of significance. Did these priests, who had the power of levitating stones, later embody in Egypt and assist in building the Great Pyramid at Gizah? Many have wondered how man could place single stones, weighing 20 tons each, to positions of great elevation, and with such precision, that one can hardly fit a razor blade between the joints.

The psychic, Betty Bethards, in her book *Atlantis* suggests how the pyramids of Egypt were built. First stones were cut from a quarry, using the energy of the third eye as a cutting tool. The third eye was located in the forehead of these advanced beings, between the eyes. Then the stone was transported above a nine-man group from the quarry to the construction site by the power of levitation. The group could levitate a stone for a distance of two miles before their mental energies would give out. Once the block arrived at the site, the same group would levitate it into its final position.

We don't have to go all the way to Egypt to admire excellent craftsmanship in stone-masonry. We have such an example right here in the United States. The late Edward Leedscalnin, an immigrant from Europe, built some marvelous stone structures at Coral Castle (28655 S. Federal Hwy, Homestead, Fla. 33030) near Miami, in the 1930's and 1940's, that have baffled the minds of many. Working all by himself, and using only ordinary tools (stone-chisels, block and tackle, and some old metal-chains) he lifted heavy stones weighing up to 28 tons, over 10 feet high. All joints are very tightly matched and perfectly square. As material he used coral, which he found on his property. As seen on the television series, "In Search of . . .," a crane operator using a modern heavy crane tried in vain to duplicate this feat. Either the cable snapped or the sides of the sharp-cornered blocks of coral chipped off. Leedscalnin often worked at night to keep away the curious. It is said he did have electricity, yet his place was not connected to a power line. Is it possible that he tapped into the magnetic currents that are around us, in the it was done on Atlantis, where generators tapped into the energy currents of the air and supplied all needs for heat, light and transportation? Leedscalnin claimed he knew how the Great Pyramid at Gizah was built, and the fruits of his labor show that he may be entitled to this claim.

Continuing the account of the Masters, in the building of Shamballa, the first task of the priests was to build a beautiful bridge connecting the mainland with the island. It was carved of the finest marble, engrained with pure gold, and contained exquisite figures of Cherubim. Adjacent to the bridge on White Island was a tree-lined avenue which led to the main temple, meant to be Sanat Kumara's residence. The main temple was built upon the highest point of the city. There were marble steps leading to it, broken by grassy terraces placed at intervals of about 12 steps. These terraces were adorned with gaily colored flowers and rainbow-hued fountains. The great door of the temple was of tremendous height. Its golden filigree work reflected the sun like a gigantic mirror. The main temple itself, as well as the remainder of the city, was built using white marble, hence the names "White Island" and "City of White."

The temple for Sanat Kumara looked similar to the Taj Mahal of modern times. It was of Cyclopean architecture. White minarets of the City pointed heavenward, and its golden-domed temples gave the impression of a gigantic fire-lotus suspended in the atmosphere. Lovely fountains adorned the front of the building.

Shamballa was not built all at once. Construction was frequently interrupted by destructive hordes, who came down from the hills, killed the builders, and destroyed their work. As soon as their physical bodies were disconnected from their etheric bodies (souls), they applied again to be quickly provided with opportunity for a new embodiment. This request was always granted. Undauntedly, for 900 years, the builders of Shamballa continued their service of love, brushed away the rubble, and started anew, sometimes even having to rebuild the very foundation of the temples.

SANAT KUMARA ENTERS SHAMBALLA

One day, working against time, (there was a Cosmic Moment beyond which the Cosmic Law would not allow the Earth any more energy, and Sanat Kumara would have to come whether Shamballa was completed or not), the city was finished.

The Lemurian Pole Star (which apparently fulfilled a function similar to today's North Star) was at its zenith, signifying this Cosmic moment, and Sanat Kumara, accompanied by three other Kumaras from Venus, entered his residence. Happy and grateful were the builders, who had endured the 900-year effort to complete Shamballa, a place so magnificent that the like of it has never been equalled at any time on Earth. They knelt in thanksgiving before God and Sanat Kumara, this forming an etheric record. Thousands of years later pilgrims entering the United States tuned into this record in establishing Thanksgiving Day.

After arriving at Shamballa, Sanat Kumara drew forth the immortal Threefold Flame of God. The concentration of that flame had never been known on the Earth before, because it represented the vibratory action of the planet Venus. A tiny thread of this flame was anchored into the heart of each of the 10 billion lifestreams belonging to Earth's evolutions, both those in embodiment, and also those out of embodiment. The crisis passed, and Earth was saved.

THE FORMING OF THE GREAT WHITE BROTHERHOOD

Next, a ways and means had to be devised whereby the natural children of the Earth and their pledged guardian spirits might be awakened to their own responsibility in creating an aura of Light for their planet to satisfy Cosmic Law, and to allow Sanat Kumara to return to his home star. Sanat Kumara prepared for this by founding the Great White Brotherhood, a united inner group of Ascended Beings. The service of this spiritual order was to teach interested students Cosmic Law, and eventually draw them into the Brotherhood. This way they would be prepared to assume, at some future time, responsibilities and positions held by volunteers from other planets.

The Great White Brotherhood is comprised of Ascended Beings who are all specialists along some particular line of spiritual service and endeavor. Their goal is to set the Earth and its evolutions free. Members of the Great White Brotherhood live only to serve God.

The first two of Earth's lifestreams to so respond were Gautama Buddha and Lord Maitreya. From this small beginning, the Brotherhood has gained in strength and numbers through the centuries.

After Sanat Kumara arrived, a priest of the Order of Zarathustra returned to mankind the knowledge of the physical fire.

Previous to the coming of Sanat Kumara there were ages when only three persons held the connection from the Earth to the Divine Realm; at one time there was only one person. That connection held the Earth in orbit.

So it was that Shamballa was completed in three

different time intervals; once or twice it was destroyed by cataclysmic action. One Master said that the final building of Shamballa was recorded in occult literature as having occurred 60,000 years ago. According to another dictation "remnants of the bridge to 'White Island' may now still be found under the shifting sands of the Gobi Desert." The desert was formed as a result of cataclysmic action, whereby the Gobi Sea was changed to a desert. When the physical buildings of Shamballa were destroyed, an etheric counterpart of Shamballa was created above it. Sanat Kumara stayed at this Etheric Retreat until 1956, when he was able to return to Venus through the efforts of students of the Light. These students, through voluntary application of the Law, had increased the Light-Quota of the Earth by constructively qualifying energy. This way they did create the necessary conditions for Sanat Kumara's return.

Let us ever be grateful to and remember the service given by Sanat Kumara, one of the greatest friends the Earth has ever known.

6 - The Lemurian Age (4,500,000 B.C.? to 200,000 B.C.)

SIZE AND LOCATION OF LEMURIA

As stated before, from the very beginning there were always several continents in existence upon the Earth's surface. So when we talk about a "Lemurian Age," this does not mean that the continent of Lemuria (sometimes called Mu), existed by itself. The reason we connect a particular age to a specific continent is, that during that particular time, its inhabitants were leaders in terms of knowledge and application of Cosmic Law and scientific achievements; hence the names "Lemurian Age" and "Atlantean Age."

Lands belonging to the gigantic continent of Lemuria included lands now under the Pacific Ocean as well as Hawaii, the Easter Islands, the Fiji Islands, Australia and New Zealand. One dictation includes lands in the Indian Ocean and Madagascar. The eastern coast of Mu extended to the area of San Diego, California.

Since it was explained by the Masters (see chapter on the "Fall of Man") that the fall of man occurred on Australia and New Zealand, this shows that these areas were above water from the very beginning.

It was stated that the Fiji Islands have been above water for at least 1.4 million years, and that Madagascar and the Baja Peninsula in Mexico have been above water for one million years.

We must conclude that the Rocky Mountains (Wyoming), Tibet, China, and Atlantis were above water 200,000 years ago, since part of the treasures of Lemuria were transferred to these locations by disciples of the Ascended Masters prior to Lemuria's sinking, which apparently happened 200,000 years ago. (See Section "The Sinking of Lemuria").

According to A.D.K. Luk, during the Lemurian Age Europe consisted of 13 states, including Switzerland, England and France. Switzerland at that time had assumed a position of leadership.

HIGHLIGHTS OF THE LEMURIAN AGE

The information given by the Masters on this subject consists, for the most part, of details concerning the size, location and sinking of Lemuria. Very little was given about highpoints of civilization and life on Lemuria.

From the sparse data that is available, it seems that after the "fall of man," the Lemurian civilization was characterized with the same up and down cycles that have been typical of recent races.

"Certain high points of this civilization occurred 800,000, 400,000, 280,000 and 200,000 years ago." When we are talking about high points, we refer to a time period in which people were willing to listen to the still, small voice within, and had a working knowledge of Cosmic Law. "The civilization of 200,000 years ago, as well as later civilizations on Atlantis, and on the Amazon River, had the knowledge and use of the Sacred Fire to the point that the flame was visible."

One might ask, how can it be that the Mu Civilization of 200,000 years ago, reached a high cultural and religious level, and then a short time later most of the continent sank? Cosmic Law requires individuals to give, at all times, a constructive response, a balance, for life and energy received. When a civilization is fortunate enough to reach a high point of accomplishment, this then is accompanied by greater assistance from above, and this greater assistance must be earned continuously, and must be balanced by a larger constructive effort. If this response is not forthcoming, the assistance from higher realms must diminish. Therefore, the higher the state of civilization a people reaches, the greater the potential for a sudden downfall.

The example of the sinking of Poseidonis, a remnant of Atlantis, may also be helpful in answering that question. The Masters stated that it was mainly during the last 500 years before the catastrophe that mankind was degraded to a very low level. This caused the ensuing chaos. Until that point, Poseidonis had achieved and maintained a level of leadership in many areas. Therefore, it is entirely possible that a similar situation existed on Mu.

"As a result of wars, great devastations took place on Mu and on Atlantis, but not on North America." Details were not provided. As a matter of fact, all of the dictations hardly ever mention any war. Apparently the Masters figured that nothing could be gained from such knowledge. Wars create destructive etheric records, and mankind should rather tune into constructive endeavors, which have a tendency to uplift.

WARNINGS

One hundred years before the sinking of the continent, the priesthood and the remaining inhabitants of Mu were warned of the potential cataclysm. The masses were advised to change their ways.

Initially there was great alarm, but when nothing immediately happened, the people and some of the priests did not heed the warning. Nearly all slipped into lethargy. The remaining priests made spiritual application through invocations for 100 years to prevent the prophesied sinking of Mu. Then they resigned themselves to the coming event. The Masters pointed out that a united priesthood could have prevented the sinking of Mu.

Just before the cataclysm, some of the temple guards transferred documents, the various flames of the temples, and other valuables to certain places that would withstand the force of the inferno. Those places were India, China, Tibet, the Rocky Mountains, and Atlantis. Djwal Kul, who later became one of the three wise men of Biblical times, participated in the safe-keeping effort by transporting certain items to Central Asia. Lord Lanto, who was then a head priest at one of the temples on Lemuria, where precipitation was successfully practiced, transported the temple flame to the Royal Teton Retreat, where it remains.

In this way the memories and the heritage of Lemuria were kept alive by a faithful few.

THE SINKING OF LEMURIA

Elohim Orion stated in 1954 that temples, cities, and entire civilizations have fallen into decay, and continents have sunk, all because peace and harmony were not sustained. Ascended Master Mary stated that spiritual arrogance destroyed the temples of Lemuria and Atlantis. She admonished the students to "keep humble in your knowledge." In another dictation it was stated, "Cataclysms come only through the destructive influence of the human, and when that is removed, there will no longer be a cause for them!"

Man's misqualified energies cause linear gas belts, which are pressure chambers located beneath the earth's surface. They are the cause of volcanic eruptions and earthquakes.

James C. Churchward's book, *The Second Book of the Cosmic Forces on Mu*, explains gas belts and gives their locations.

The Ascended Master Saint Germain, in a dictation given in 1936 on the Hawaiian Islands, answered Mr. Ballard's great desire for some authentic information as to the origin of the islands. He explained that before the sinking of Mu there was a long mountain range traversing the larger part of the continent in an almost west-east direction. The western limit of the range was located a bit more to the north than the eastern extremity of the range. There was another mountain chain running in a north-south direction. These two ranges were the highest ones on the continent.

Continuing Saint Germain's account, "200,000 years ago, at the time of the great cataclysm, these mountain ranges were raised to their greatest height, namely, to a range of 18,000 to 20,000 ft. above water. The range going almost east and west was on a powerful double gas belt. This was largely responsible for Lemuria's sinking. After it sank, the mountains remained 10,000 to 15,000 feet above sea level." From the preceding it appears that the Mu catastrophe happened 200,000 years ago.

James C. Churchward explains the action of a pressure chamber on a mountain. The internal pressure of the underground pocket forces the top of a mountain higher and higher, to a point where the walls of the mountain get too thin to counteract the expansion pressure, and the whole mountain explodes. Its remainder then collapses within itself.

Saint Germain stated that today's geysers and hot springs in Yellowstone Park are situated on a gas belt. If it were not for this activity, the surface of the earth would be torn apart by the underground pressure. Therefore, the geysers and springs act as a safety valve.

In the book, *Unveiled Mysteries*, it is stated that a cataclysm occurred which tore the surface of the earth until all collapsed within itself. Mu sank below the waves of what is now the Pacific Ocean. It will rise again.

According to the Ascended Master Cuzco, Mu submerged overnight, with a population of 60 million people.

A dictation of Lord Himalaya in 1959 confirms that Mu went down overnight. This dictation provides further interesting details. The continent sank so quietly that nearly everybody was totally unaware of what was happening. Practically all were sleeping during the episode. There were no unusual weather conditions; the sky was blue. What happened to the remaining temple priests? Like captains on a sinking ship, they kept their posts, and fearless to the end, they sang as they went down. The melody they sang was the same that is known today as "Auld Lang Syne." The idea behind this action was that every horrifying experience leaves a deep scar on the etheric body, which sometimes takes several embodiments to heal. Through the action of the priests staying together and singing, much fear was mitigated, and a certain amount of harmony was maintained. This way the damage to the etheric bodies was held to a minimum.

According to A.D.K. Luk, Europe sank with Mu, except for the top of the Swiss Alps, which remained above water.

The Mu catastrophe was accompanied by a shift in the poles. Such a shift occurs at every major cataclysm.

The earliest cataclysm, according to my research of the dictations of the Masters, occurred 200,000 years ago. A.D.K. Luk lists cataclysms occurring 800,000 and 1,000,000 years ago. (*Law of Life*, Vol 1, p.240).

7 - The Atlantean Age (500,000 B.C. to 10,000 B.C.)

SIZE AND LOCATION OF ATLANTIS

We can consider ourselves fortunate, indeed, that the Masters left us some tangible details concerning the rise and fall of several civilizations during the Atlantean Age. No longer do we have to rely only upon mythology, legends, psychic testimony, allegories, and veiled or even incorrect information presented by the Masters, who were severely limited by the occult law as it applied to the Earth. The Masters said that the type of information released after 1930 had not been permitted to be given for 12,000 years.

The Atlantean continent originally consisted of a solid land mass, reaching from Central America to Europe. According to one dictation, "Europe then was part of Atlantis." Cuba, the Madeira Islands, and the Azores were also part of it. There is also some indication that a section of the United States was considered part of Atlantis, because the Masters labeled temples located on its east coast as "Atlantean Temples." There were also other continents on the Earth's surface during the Atlantean Age.

An Atlantean civilization was first mentioned by the Masters as having existed 500,000 years ago. The last remnant of Atlantis sank 10,000 B.C. Therefore, this publication considers that the Atlantean Age took place from 500,000 B.C. to 10,000 B.C..

ATLANTEAN AGE CIVILIZATIONS

The Atlantean culture reached one of its heights 500,000 years ago. The people of that age had achieved great illumination, understanding, and oneness with the God-Presence. They knew the power of radiation, and the importance of vibratory action that passed through the bodies of individuals.

At that time, Long Island, an island near New York City, was considered holy ground, and it was entirely dedicated to the priesthood. No one, except the priesthood, was allowed on the island. Through the purity and constructive activity of the priests, Long Island became the most highly-magnetized center of spiritual currents on the Earth's surface at that time. It was not advisable for anyone to step on the island, for it was like touching a high tension wire.

After the sinking of Mu, 200,000 years ago, its priesthood soon thereafter embodied on Atlantis. Endowed with the gift of consecutive consciousness (the memory of previous embodiments), they drew those lifestreams around them who assisted them during former Golden Ages on Mu. Therefore, soon after the Mu age, the Atlantean culture flourished.

In several respects, the technology of the various Atlantean civilizations was superior to that of today. Unlimited energy necessary for lighting, heating, propulsion of boats, transportation, and airships was drawn forth from the atmosphere, and received and transmitted through power boxes, measuring two feet by two feet by three feet. By means of its airships, Atlantis stayed in touch with all part of the globe.

The Atomic Accelerator, a device accelerating the vibratory action of the four lower bodies, was used as a healing, purifying agent.

The superior technology, coupled with a good understanding of Cosmic Law, enabled the Atlantean civilization to maintain a position of leadership which endured for thousands of years, up to the time of the sinking of its last remnant, the isle of Poseidonis. During its heights, Atlantis was considered a worldwide empire.

The Masters cited the Sahara, Gobi, and Texas civilizations as superior civilizations. Those reached their peak about 70,000 years ago. They will be discussed in more detail later in this book.

About 28,000 years ago some civilizations must have reached high points, because the Masters stated that at that time there were groups of beings whose natural radiance illuminated everything, wherever they went. They also stated that this accomplishment is possible for students today.

Last in our chronology, the civilizations of Meru and Poseidonis need to be mentioned. These civilizations reached high points in the time periods of 12,000 B.C. to 10,000 B.C., and from 12,000 to 10,500 B.C. respectively. For reasons explained later, I assume that the Meru and Poseidonis civilizations were both destroyed by the cataclysm that occurred about 10,000 B.C.

ATLANTEAN TEMPLES

The Atlantean temples were a focal point for pilgrims coming from all parts of the globe, including those from different continents. They were given beautiful accommodations.

Some of the priests had achieved the ability to levitate. Thus, they were able to attend the conventions at certain main temples by levitating back and forth from their homes.

The Masters spoke of the following main temples:

1) "Early Atlantean Age": (age not given)
   - Temple of Purification by Violet Fire, near Cuba
   - Temple of Faith and Protection, Philadelphia
   - Temple of Power and Protection, Harrisburg, Pennsylvania
   - Temple of the Comfort of the Holy Spirit, Long Island, N.Y.
   - Temple of Divine Love, New Bedford, Massachusetts
   - Temple of Cosmic Christ Truth, Middle West, U.S.A. (Denver?), Pallas Athena was High Priestess at this temple. Jade Temple, Chicago

2) Later Age (age not given)
   - Temples of the Sun, New York City. There were 12 temples around a central temple. The central temple contained the Liberty Flame.
   - Temple of the Seven Elohim, San Francisco, later destroyed by a black magician.
   - Temple of the Angels, Los Angeles
   - Temple of Archangel Chamuel, Blue Ridge Mountains, Virginia

Temple of the Sacred Heart, location not given

Nada, who made her ascension 2,700 years ago, served at the Temple of Divine Love near New Bedford. Here healing work was done by directing light rays. This included sending rays to patients present at the temple, as well as to others not present (called absent treatment of healing).

During an early time period of the Atlantean Age, Divine Beings, Archangels and angels walked and talked with man. This was done for the spiritual uplift of the people, just as it was before the fall of man, demonstrating that renting the veil is an ever-present possibility.

Among the White Order of the priesthood (the Great White Brotherhood), were priests and priestesses of the Order of Archangel Zadkiel. They served in the Temple of Purification by Violet Fire. The Temple of Purification was of circular design and around it were located seven smaller temples. The temples were situated adjacent to the present Cuba, which at that time was part of the continent of Atlantis. From the golden dome of each temple arose a living, visible violet flame which could be seen within a radius of 1,000 miles. Saint Germain, not yet ascended at that time, served as one of the priests in the Central Temple.

The Order of Archangel Zadkiel was the heart-center of maintaining God's plan for Earth. The activity of the Seventh Ray was naturally developed through instruction and training of lifestreams in the power of invocation (decreeing), and in holding the attention upon God, the universal I AM Presence. Through the power of that sustained attention, the mercy of God was magnetized until it became a tremendous force for good. Rhythm of invocation, constancy of devotion to the magnetization, sustenance and expansion of the

Violet Fire through meditation, contemplation, songs, and decrees were the fundamental teachings of the temples of Archangel Zadkiel.

All other priests of the White Order were fully aware of this focus, and often came themselves to bathe in the purifying essence of this flame. They also sent their chelas to Lord Zadkiel's Temple, so the effluvia of discord that was growing upon Atlantis might be dislodged from their consciousness. These students left the temple purified and revitalized, eager and willing to serve in their own temples to preserve the Divine Will and the kingdom of righteousness on Earth.

ATLANTEAN WARS AND CATACLYSMS

Introduction

During the Atlantean Age, civilizations reached great heights, but there were many low points as well. Numerous wars took place on both sides of North America, namely on Lemuria and on Atlantis. In Europe, which at that time was part of Atlantis, mankind was determined to destroy one another.

Saint Germain stated that the human ungoverned is more vicious than the jungle! Three times a most poisonous, destructive, gas-substance was used. It wiped out entire populations of cities, leaving only the buildings intact. The physical bodies of the people were destroyed in a few minutes.

The Ascended Masters provided us with the description of only one war, namely the war near today's Cuba. Descriptions of wars tend to focus our attention upon destructive etheric records. Energy follows thought, and the imperfect use of energy does not help our freedom. The Masters gave us a detailed description of the war near Cuba because it illustrates the ever on-going battle between the forces of good and evil — white and black magic. In addition, the details explain the cause of the future sinking of a portion of the Atlantean Continent.

Forces of Light and Forces of Darkness

Before discussing the great battle between the forces of light and darkness that took place on Atlantis, it would seem of advantage to deal with some general basic concepts of Cosmic Law, as they apply to dark forces. The following illustration may help.

To understand those forces, let us begin by examining a typical chela (dedicated student) on the path. Under the action of the Law, as it applied prior to 1930, the chela was admitted to a retreat after reaching a certain state of purification and enlightenment. Here he was placed under the general supervision of a master.

Often, especially in the beginning, the chela was left to his own heart's prompting, as to how to proceed. As the months and years went by, he was taught a point of law here and there. He was asked to pass many tests and many initiations.

Frustrated by the severity of the tests, the slow process of receiving additional instruction, having little contact with the master in the beginning, and discouraged by the austere surroundings, many chelas left the retreat, some never to return. Some of the chelas who left, harbored feelings of rebellion, discouragement, and resentment. A few of them degraded to the point where they became prey for "black magicians," also called "members of the black order." (Edgar Cayce calls them "sons of Belial".) The black order gained the confidence of such students by carefully and skillfully duplicating the activity of the "White Order," offering them less difficult and faster progress, and appealing to their ego by such means as offering a certificate of accomplishment or a degree. They also came up with a counterpart to the "Elixir of Life." An elixir is a drink prepared by a master to refresh and rejuvenate the student in mind and body. The black order countered this by coming up with alcoholic drinks.

Once he became a follower, the student, through fear, was held loyal to the teachings of the black magicians, whose intent was, and is to destroy the Light wherever they can find it. This type of action has been going on for 680,000 years, and at times there were regular schools of black magic.

What can the student's former master do? Very little, if anything. He knows that free will is an attribute given to man by God; therefore, the master cannot interfere. To make things worse, the master now has to transmute some of the karma of the student's fall; that is, the teacher is made personally responsible for the student's transgressions. It is no wonder that personal instruction by a master is never imparted lightly. It has to be earned by the chela.

What kind of power does a black magician have over a student of Ascended Master teaching? None — provided the student protects himself on a daily basis, and keeps his harmony. Then he has nothing to fear. Saint Germain said to Mr. Ballard, "You will be protected, IF you keep your harmony!"

According to the eyewitness, many "I AM students" of the 1930's had encounters with "black magicians," who ran rampant until 1937. The knowledge and application of the Violet Flame and the protective pillar of Light were most helpful to the students. All of us who consider ourselves "students on the path" owe a great deal of gratitude to the early students under Mr. Ballard. They had to bear the brunt of the battle. Because of their daily invocations, the most vicious foci of the dark forces were destroyed, and most of the black magicians, especially those operating within the United States, were rendered ineffective. However, some dark forces remain. Therefore, wise is the student who daily protects himself and keeps his harmony.

With this explanation behind us, we are now ready to proceed with the subject at hand.

The Battle Near Cuba

"The battle plan of the black magicians was to draw fearful, skeptical, disappointed, and rebellious individuals to them," and to attack the central bulwark of the opponent, namely the "White Order," located at Archangel Zadkiel's "Temple of Purification by Violet Fire." This temple was situated near today's Cuba, on Atlantis. Thus started one of the greatest battles between the forces of light and darkness the Earth has ever known.

In time, the battle plan of the black magicians succeeded. Gradually and secretly, most of the priests of the "White Order" aligned themselves with the "black order." Through fear, the followers of the "black order" were held loyal to its teachings. Few remained sincerely affiliated with the "White Order," and because of lack of support by a sufficient amount of followers, Archangel Zadkiel had to withdraw from having outer contact with the priests of the temple. As a consequence of insufficient invocation (decreeing) by the priesthood the violet flame no longer was visible.

The disloyalty by the priesthood, together with the malpractice of some priests in aligning themselves with the dark forces, made possible the sinking of a great continent. Its spiritual anchorage having been destroyed, the "Temple of Purification by Violet Fire" sank beneath the Atlantic with a major portion of the Atlantean Continent. Before its sinking the temple was etheralized. It is still pulsating in the ethers near the island of Cuba today.

The "black order" could not, however, erase the memory of the Violet Fire of mercy and compassion from the etheric consciousness of those who served in the temples. One such priest who kept this consciousness is the Ascended Master Saint Germain, now Chohan (Lord) of the Seventh Ray. He, as well as others, remembered the glory of Archangel Zadkiel's temple, and the tremendous service it had rendered to the people of Atlantis. The Law of Life does not allow any force of evil to destroy the memory of the glory of a former Golden Age.

THE BREAKUP OF THE ATLANTEAN CONTINENT

When the forces of darkness had sufficiently influenced the consciousness of a large majority of the people on Atlantis in disobeying God and following the rebellious way of the destructive use of free will, and when there was insufficient constructive use of energy by the priesthood, the Cosmic Law decreed that Atlantis no longer justified its right to exist.

The first cataclysm during the time period under consideration (500,000 B.C. to 10,000 B.C.) occurred 200,000 years ago, and has already been reported under the section, "The Lemurian Age." Since this cataclysm tore apart a large portion of the Earth's surface, it is possible that portions of Atlantis sank also at that time.

The second major cataclysm of this time period took place 80,000 years ago. It must have been a world-wide catastrophe of devastating impact, because the Masters stated that the cataclysm of 80,000 years ago changed the colors of the Earth, and for the first time the colors red and black became known to mankind. The Masters explained in another dictation that these colors have a tendency to lower the vibrations of the individual by appealing to the lower senses.

During this cataclysm the Golden Gate and San Francisco Harbor came into existence. (The Golden Gate is a narrow waterway between the San Francisco peninsula and the mainland to the north. The waterway is now bridged by the Golden Gate Bridge.) There were no subsequent changes to the earth's surface in the San Francisco area. The seven hills of San Francisco have existed for over 80,000 years. At that time the city was known as the City of the Seven Hills.

The area now known as the state of Texas was raised during this cataclysm. It was below the surface of the water prior to this event.

During several cataclysms the tearing apart of the Earth's surface was re-experienced, and piece by piece, various portions of the giant continent of Atlantis submerged beneath the ocean. This process took place over a time period of thousands of years. Finally, only the island of Poseidonis, a central and small remnant of the original continent, remained. As part of cataclysmic action, lands west and east of

Poseidonis had sunk beneath the ocean. The lands that submerged included portions located in the vicinity of today's Cuba.

Poseidonis, when still part of the larger continent, had been the heart-center of the then-known civilized world. The Masters protected this part of Atlantis in order to continue important activities on Poseidonis, and to use it as a central focus in completing certain unfinished work.

A.D.K. Luk states, (*Law of Life and Teaching by Divine Beings*, p. 164), that the sinking of Atlantis started by its being separated from Europe and North America; it became a separate continent. The British Isles remained above water. Then, from time to time, portions of Atlantis sank, until only the island of Poseidonis, reaching from the vicinity of Greenland to the Azores, was left.

The Final Atlantean cataclysm took place about 10,000 B.C. At that time Poseidonis, the last remaining fragment of Atlantis, was submerged. This event will be further described under the sections, "The Meru Civilization," and "The Poseidonis Civilization."

THE GOLDEN AGE OF THE SAHARA EMPIRE

Introduction

Thousands of years ago there existed a civilization that extended from the present Sahara Desert (its westerly boundary), across the entire width of Africa, continuing east across Asia, all the way to the Himalayan Mountains. This civilization was called the "Sahara Empire," and it reached such a high level of attainment that the term "Golden Age" has been attributed to this time period.

The Sahara Desert was fertile land at that time. There were many streams of water, and the entire area enjoyed abundant moisture and a semi-tropical climate. The Nile, as it is today, resembles the streams of that period. The following description of the civilization and prevailing conditions pertain to the year 68,000 B.C., when the Sahara Kingdom reached its apex.

The Sahara Kingdom

In the midst of the Sahara empire was the capital, famous throughout the world for its splendor. The executive buildings were located in the center of the capital, upon a slight elevation, and from this hub, the city, itself, extended equally in every direction. The name of the city was known as "the City of the Sun." The domes of many buildings were covered with sheets of pure gold, and the interiors decorated with jewels. The gold and the jewels were precipitated directly from the One Eternal Substance.

The king-emperor, then unascended, was the Master now known to us as Saint Germain. His empire was a living example of perfection; there has never been anything on Earth since that time which has ever approached such heights. For hundreds of years this perfection was sustained, and there was no need for an army and navy of any kind.

Saint Germain was assisted by a Council of fourteen Ascended Masters, two working on each of the seven rays. The government, itself, consisted of seven departments, which controlled the activities of science, industry and art. Each department head worked directly with the council, and therefore was attuned at all times to the divine plan. Everybody served for the good of all.

The Downfall

The downfall of this civilization sounds like a familiar story. We find the same inner causes already given for the "fall of man," the Lemurian civilization, and Atlantis. They were the same causes that later destroyed the last remnant of Atlantis, called Poseidonis.

The downward trend started when people turned their attention away from God, to themselves. The Sahara Civilization became emmeshed in sense gratification. They were ungrateful for the blessings nature pours out, and for life itself. There was misuse of energy, and the inhabitants became selfish, all of which created destructive conditions. God, the giver of all life-energy, expects right use of that energy, so it may bless the rest of creation with harmonious activity. Without such right use of energy, a civilization can no longer be sustained under the divine plan, and so it collapses.

The king-emperor, foreseeing what was to happen, called his council and their staffs to his palace. An elaborate banquet was held, all food and drink being precipitated. Five hundred seventy-six people were present.

An Ascended Master appeared out of nowhere and addressed the audience. He explained that because of the downfall of the civilization, the king and his family had to be taken away. He also predicted that a prince, now approaching the border of the kingdom, would take over the rule of the empire. After the Master had finished, he slowly disappeared from sight.

Seven days after the banquet, the King-Emperor left, and was seen no more.

A visiting prince of a lesser-developed country

arrived shortly thereafter, and discovering the condition of the empire, installed himself as ruler. He found no opposition.

Two thousand years later (66,000 B.C.), most of the empire became barren land. The streams dried up, and desolation reigned everywhere, the result of mankind's discord.

Thereafter (no date given) followed a great cataclysm, forming an inland sea, where the Sahara Desert now lies. The cataclysm that submerged Poseidonis about 10,000 B.C. later drained this sea, and part of the original Sahara Empire became what is known today as the Sahara Desert.

OTHER CIVILIZATIONS, 68,000 B.C.

The Gobi civilization coexisted with the Sahara civilization. [Since the Sahara civilization extended to the Himalayas, the Gobi civilization may have bordered it.] Both reached a high point of development at approximately the same time, and suffered the same fate, namely, the apex of attainment was not ended by a cataclysm, but both civilizations were taken over by primitive hordes.

A highly-developed civilization came forth in Texas at the same time as the Sahara civilization, 70,000 years ago.

The Masters stated that the procedure of systematic preservation of records started as early as 68,000 B.C., which would cover the time-period of these civilizations.

No information was given by the Masters about the Great Pyramid at Gizah. Therefore, I am unable to comment upon whether or not ancient records are stored in this structure or in its vicinity, as Edgar Cayce claims.

THE MERU CIVILIZATION

Life Along the Amazon River

From 12,000 B.C. to 10,000 B.C. there existed a civilization in South America which reached a great height of accomplishment. It co-existed with the civilization of Poseidonis, the last remnant of the large continent of Atlantis, and was a child of Atlantean culture and attainment.

South America at that time was called Meru, after God Meru, who is the Manu of the sixth rootrace, and whose retreat is near Lake Titicaca.

The civilization centered along the Amazon River, the Madeira River, and the Jurua River, and extended in an east-west direction from the Amazon delta to approximately seventy degrees west longitude, to the easterly border of Peru and Colombia.

The name "Amazon" means "boat destroyer," referring to the cataclysm that occurred about 10,000 B.C., which severely damaged South America and sank Poseidonis. The river at that time was navigable, extending from Lake Titicaca to the Atlantic Ocean. A canal was built from the Pacific Ocean to Lake Titicaca. This connection with the Amazon formed an entire waterway between the two oceans. The river was much deeper than it is today.

Near the mouth of the Amazon there were wide, beautiful falls. Between the falls and the seacoast, originally about ten miles south of the river, there existed a city of importance. It was buried during the cataclysm that destroyed the Meru civilization. This city rests now fifty feet below the surface of the earth.

The mouth of the Amazon was widened many miles during the cataclysm that occurred 12,000 years ago. An obelisk of imperishable metal, covered with hieroglyphs of the former age, marked the highest point of the city. The obelisk was originally 60 feet high.

The capital of the empire, which was its religious center, was located near the Madeira River. The second city of importance was located near the Jurua River. It was a center of commerce, and many governmental buildings were located here. Also, it was the center of the jewelry industry. Many precious stones were cut and polished here. As a result of the cataclysm, this city suffered the same fate as the city near the mouth of the Amazon.

The capital was laid out in a series of concentric circles, the innermost of which measured four miles in diameter. The area of this innermost circle was used to accommodate the executive buildings of the empire. Business streets went out from this innermost circle like spokes from the hub of a wheel. All business streets were paved and constructed eighteen inches to twenty-four inches below the surrounding ground. They were flooded every morning and washed thoroughly clean before the activities of the day began.

Three miles from the innermost circle there were landscaped streets which functioned as scenic roads for pleasure drives. Therefore, the business activities did not interfere with the beauty and convenience of the drives.

Almost all of the buildings contained top floors which featured adjustable domes. These were constructed in four sections, and could be arranged as sleeping quarters or for purposes of entertainment.

The climate was semi-tropical, the days being always warm and comfortable. Extreme temperatures were unknown, and at night there was a cooling breeze from the mountains.

The Capitol, itself, was a large structure surfaced with cream-colored marble. Its floor was made of green-colored stone tile.

A gigantic temple called "God's Living Temple to Man" was the spiritual center of the capital city and the entire civilization. It had a seating capacity of ten thousand people. In the center of the temple stood a square column, twenty feet high. Upon this stood a crystal globe, two feet in diameter. A soft, self luminous white light was contained within. Despite its softness, it was so intensely luminous that the entire temple was brilliantly lighted by it. This focus of light was drawn and placed in the temple by a Cosmic Master as a sustaining and life-giving activity for the people. The crystal globe sent forth not only light, but also energy and power, forming one of the basic means of sustaining the activities of the Meru civilization.

Energy necessary for light, heat and power for propulsion was also generated and transmitted by instrument-like power boxes. If used for propulsion they were attached to the vehicle used. Seven different types of these energy-transmitting boxes were in use. The boxes had a volume of two feet by two feet by three feet. They had the capability of gathering the energy currents existing in the atmosphere. These currents of electricity were of a higher, finer type than that which is used now. They could be affected through thought force, but could be controlled through mechanical means as well.

Saint Germain reported another achievement in the field of technology. Certain metals were combined with glass through a fusing process, to make the product strong as steel and imperishable. [Perhaps the obelisk of the aforementioned city near the mouth of the Amazon was made of this material.]

The people living in Meru had golden hair with pink and white complexions. The men were about six feet three inches in height, the women averaging five feet ten. All had eyes of a beautiful violet-blue color. The race expressed a serene, calm intelligence.

The name of the emperor was Casimir Poseidon, an Ascended Master who was a direct descendant of the Mighty Ascended Master Rulers of Atlantis. His crown consisted of a simple band of gold with a large diamond in the center of the forehead. His heavy golden hair hung full to his shoulders. "Casimir Poseidon was greatly loved by his people, and his memory was kept alive for many centuries in myth and fable."

Preservation of Records

The records of this civilization were preserved by the Ascended Masters. They are kept for future use in metal boxes which are two feet long, fourteen inches wide, and six inches deep. These records were made by writing upon sheets of gold with a stylus. At one time the records were kept at "God's Living Temple to Man." The original, or a copy of it, is now kept at the Teton Retreat. One day, in the future, the records and the accomplishments of the Meru civilization will be revealed to the outer world.

The Warning

Shortly before the capital just described was buried, it reached the height of its glory, and the Great Cosmic Master who initially drew the Light by which it was developed and sustained, appeared for the last time to the empire. He foretold of an unavoidable cataclysm and announced that this was his last appearance. He gave no time period for the cataclysm. Those who wished to save themselves were instructed to leave and directed where to go. The warning was given that the catastrophe would be sudden and complete. After finishing this prophesy, his body faded rapidly from sight. To the dismay of the people, the pedestal and the crystal globe holding the Eternal Light disappeared with him.

The Cataclysm

After a year had passed, the memory of the prophecy faded. Since nothing unusual happened, the population's anxiety passed away. Doubt began to appear as to the reality of the coming cataclysm.

Casimir Poseidon, and those more spiritually advanced, left the area and began to take up residence in the western part of the United States. Here they remained until the cataclysm was over. Before leaving, the emperor had sealed his palace and the temple in which the before-described sphere of light had been maintained.

The remaining people in Meru became more and more skeptical and rebellious. One person attempted to force an entrance to the sealed temple. He fell lifeless at its door.

Near the end of the fifth year following the prophecy the sun darkened at noon, and an awful terror filled the atmosphere. At sunset, terrific quakes shook the earth and demolished all buildings. Chaos was everywhere. "Before the coming of dawn the great destructive powers had done their work."

"The entire continent of Meru, now called South America, lost its equilibrium. It tilted and rolled to the east, submerging the entire eastern coast for a distance of 160 feet." The coast remained in this position for several years. Then it gradually righted itself to within 60 feet of the original position. No subsequent changes in elevation have occurred since.

Thus, another civilization of splendid achievement came to an abrupt close. Master Saint Germain explained how a civilization, beautiful and perfect in every way, could suffer the tragedy of a destructive cataclysm. When a group of mankind is fortunate enough to come under the radiation of a Great Master of Light, in return as a balance, a continuous, conscious effort is needed to be made by mankind to understand Cosmic Law and to willingly work in harmonious cooperation with it. According to God's Law, if a group of mankind has been taught the way of mastery and has been reminded lifetime after lifetime of their divine birthright and their balancing effort is not forthcoming, the Masters of Light must withdraw their sustaining power.

Thoughts and feelings of hate, anger, resentment of any kind, and revenge are recorded by all of the elemental (nature) beings. When such misqualified energy has accumulated to a certain pressure, a self-generating and self-purifying force within nature rises and throws off all that disagrees with the "Law of the One." Thus, the qualities recorded return to their source, individual man, in the form of cataclysms, by means of the four elements of nature. Thus a cataclysm is nature's way of relieving, purifying and shaking herself free of the contamination of human, discordant thoughts and feelings, and returning to her pristine condition.

Students of Ascended Master teaching can do much to relieve the discordant conditions of nature caused by mankind's previous misuse of energy. There is a great need to transmute the misqualified energy gathered in the gas belts. This is done through decreeing in groups or singly. ("Thou shalt decree a thing and it shall be done unto thee," Job: 22,28.) The power of the spoken word is most effective.

THE POSEIDONIS CIVILIZATION

Location

Poseidonis was the name of an island located in the middle of the Atlantic Ocean. It was the last surviving remnant of the original continent of Atlantis.

This small remnant of the originally very large continent of Atlantis is often confused with Atlantis itself. Even Plato, who, according to the Rosicrucian Order, was a member of a secret mystery school, called the island "Atlantis." Sometimes this difficulty in separating and distinguishing between the two terms applies also to the material given by the Ascended Masters. Fortunately, by reading carefully each word that is given on this subject, and comparing the different dictations, it is possible in most cases to separate the material into the earlier Atlantean times and the Poseidonis Civilization, which existed at the same time as the Meru Civilization. Both the Meru Civilization and the Poseidonis Civilization reached their apex during the time period from 12,000 B.C. to 10,000 B.C.

To the best of my knowledge, the Masters did not give the exact location of Poseidonis other than to say that it occupied a central portion of Atlantis, and to say that the Azores and Madeira Islands were part of the highest mountain ranges of Poseidonis.

A.D.K. Luk states that Poseidonis reached from south

of Greenland to the Azores. W. Scott-Elliot in his book, *The Story of Atlantis and the Lost Lemuria*, shows Poseidonis at about the same location.

Life on Poseidonis

Fourteen thousand years ago Poseidonis reached a high state of attainment with regard to knowledge of Cosmic Law and scientific achievements. A great Master of Light was at the head of its government. Its state of accomplishment was maintained until about 10,500 B.C., when the decline of the civilization began, culminating in the catastrophe that occurred around 10,000 B.C.

During the height of the Poseidonis civilization, there was a province where an attempt was made to bring forth a nation of Ascended Masters. The people living in this area were able to precipitate many things they needed from universal substance, including food and clothing. They sat at their table and the food they required appeared in front of them. The consuming activity of the Three-fold Flame (the flame referred to may be the Violet Flame), was visible to all. After having completed its service, the physical body was placed in this flame and it disappeared instantly. [Since flames were only kept at temples and maintained there by the priests, I believe this ceremony took place in temples.]

Technology was very much advanced. The Poseidonis civilization had world-wide contact through airships. Among other places, they traveled to Yellowstone Park (Wyoming, U.S.A.), and Meru. The air transportation of today in many respects is crude and primitive compared to theirs.

The richest gold mine the world has ever known

existed in Yellowstone Park. It was under the control of the Poseidonis government, and much of its wealth was used for experimental and research purposes in chemistry and other fields of natural science. The word "Yellowstone" originated from a mine in the area which contained beautiful yellow diamonds. Advanced rock drilling techniques were used in the operation of the Yellowstone mines.

The Poseidonis civilization also was able to generate energy necessary for light, heat, power, and propulsion by gathering, concentrating and transmitting currents located in the surrounding atmosphere.

Warnings

Before every major cataclysm, great efforts are made by the Masters to acquaint the people with the truth. At the time of the sinking of Poseidonis, only five hundred out of sixty million people gave credence to the words of truth. That was not enough to hold the balance.

Five years before Poseidonis sank, the Masters alerted the people as to the coming events. [This dictation checks with the five-year warning given to the Meru civilization. Both messages were given by different channels, about 28 years apart.]

Ascended Beings and Cosmic Messengers from many realms came and spoke through the priesthood and the oracles. At first the people listened to their words, and the idea was entertaining for a while. It was something new and different, and it was exciting. Then, when nothing happened for two years after the warnings, the people went back to their pursuits of so-called happiness. The Masters said that the people of Poseidonis lost faith in the priests of the true White Order, and that action severed the anchor to the island.

The Exodus

The Ascended Beings preserved buildings, entire cities, records, formulas and whatever they wished to keep by hermetically sealing them at the bottom of the Atlantic. They will bring them forth in the new age just ahead, revealing the truth of Atlantis' perfection to all.

The high priests of the temples were notified by the spiritual hierarchy to gather all the priceless treasures from the temples in which they officiated, and to load them into the vessels anchored in the harbors. Thus, the preparation for the exodus of the members of the White Order and their followers began.

Quietly and unhurriedly, the guardians of the Atlantean Age prepared for the final hour when they would be required to leave their beloved Poseidonis. Every leader was given sealed orders containing the destination of his boat. Each destination was a pre-selected haven of safety, which would either not be affected by the cataclysm at all, or at best, very little. In this manner, the truth and knowledge of Ascended Master Teaching was preserved for generations yet to come.

The priests' preparations included taking the flames from the altars and carrying them and sacred documents, containing the content of many conferences, to places of safety.

Those priests and chelas who remained true to the Light were made aware of the date when Poseidonis was to sink. At a certain pre-arranged hour, at night, the followers of the White Order loaded their boats with those temple treasures that they were able to wrest from the hands of the greedy priesthood. One hundred sailboats, equipped with oars, were manned. The boats carried forty volunteers each, including one priest per boat.

Upon leaving the shore, the leader of each boat opened the sealed orders. These documents contained the destiny of each boat. The priest, Hilarion, (who later was Paul, one of Jesus' disciples) was asked to carry the Flame of Truth across the Atlantic Ocean, through the Mediterranean, into Greece. The priest, Serapis Bey, and his group was to carry the Ascension Flame to Luxor, Egypt. Those who guarded the Flame of Liberty were directed to carry it to southern France. It was the task of the boats to arrive at a place of safety before the ocean would be churned into a boiling sea by the cataclysmic action, that no boat could survive.

"Of the one hundred boats that left Poseidonis, only ten arrived. Time and karmic conditions were such that the Cosmic Moment could not wait the arrival of the vessels at their locations, if they were delayed beyond a certain date, for any reason."

The treasures of Poseidonis were taken to different parts of the globe. Records were taken to Egypt, Tibet, China and other parts of the Far East. Some of the Atlantean records later found their way to the library in Alexandria, where ultimately most of them suffered destruction by fire. The records not carried to Alexandria have remained intact. These will come forth in the near future, when the viciousness, bigotry, and intolerance of the orthodox mind is dissolved to a point where they will not meet with destruction.

As mentioned before, ten of the boats leaving Poseidonis safely reached their destinations.

1) One boat, under the direction of Serapis Bey

arrived at Luxor.

2) One boat, under the direction of Hilarion arrived at Crete.
3) One boat, under the direction of Paul the Venetian arrived in southern France.
4) At least one boat, sailing westward, arrived in Mexico.
5) At least one boat, sailing westward, arrived in Peru.
6) At least one boat, sailing westward, arrived at the Easter Islands.
7) At least one boat, sailing westward, arrived in Asia.

Serapis Bey and his men reached their destination seconds before the Nile overflowed.

Hilarion and his group arrived safely at Crete, which at that time was connected to the mainland of Greece. Hilarion established the Flame of Truth there. This focus was later used to bring forth the Temple of Truth at Crete, and the Oracles of Delphi in Greece. Subsequent earth changes, after the Poseidonis catastrophe, disconnected Crete from the mainland.

The Ascended Master Serapis Bey gave two separate eyewitness accounts to the students about His voyage to Luxor. Because of their historic significance, they are repeated here, as originally given.

"When the final island of Atlantis was about to sink beneath the waves, the priesthood who had remained true to the Spiritual Hierarchy endeavored to reach the consciousness of the people and warn them of the impending cataclysmic changes. Novelty appeals to the outer mind, and for a time it was a subject of conversation and considerable interest, but the sustained enthusiasms and interests of the people soon determined the aspirants, the servers, the chelas from the dilettantes, and as the years went by, the priesthood became hard, arrogant, superior, so versed in the Law that they closed in a mental shell their consciousness from the pressures of inspiration and from the Christ message which comes like the dove, humbly, simply and unadorned. In this spiritual arrogance the priesthood swayed the masses, and those who represented the true spiritual order were very few.

"Those of us who did remain true to the Light were informed when it was time for the sinking of the continent. At a certain hour, on a certain night we loaded our boats with all the beautiful treasures from our Temples, those that we were able to wrest from the hands of the greedy priesthood, with a prayer in our hearts and the faithful few in our boats, we sailed across the Atlantic and the Pacific to many lands."

"None of us knew where we were going until we opened the sealed orders, after we had left the shore. We knew there was a timing, an element to be considered because the sinking of a continent vitally affects the mighty oceans, and we were in small barks which tossed like chips on the waves of the sea.

"We found on opening our orders that we were destined for Egypt. The 40 of us concentrating our prayer force, faith, physical energies and our endurance spelled ourselves off day and night, rowing to assist the sails, each trying to meet that deadline not so much interested in the survival of our bodies, but interested in getting our cargo, the embers of the Ascension Flame, which was the spiritual heritage from Atlantis entrusted to us, on dry land before our boat was overwhelmed by the rising sea. And we did! We sailed up the Nile and when we landed in the region of Luxor, we carried with us in a golden brazier, through rain, wind and storm, a living flame, heart of the Ascension Temple on Atlantis, to plant at Luxor. With our own bodies we cradled that Flame. Each one of us breathing the flame of our hearts within It and breathing the breath from our lips upon It, and the prayers of our souls and spirits kept It alive for that hour, when we landed. How grateful our hearts were that there was even an ember. Around that Flame of the Ascension we knelt and as we did, the Earth trembled and the mighty Nile swelled over its banks. I admit the tears fell, as Poseidonis, the heart of Atlantis, the home that we had known, and the temples, the magnificence of which has not yet come forth again since that day, our loved ones, our families, passed beneath the waves into the heart of the sea."

"We spelled each other off at the oars, rowing against time, knowing that a Cosmic moment waits for no weariness of flesh, no doubt of mind, no fear in the feelings, nor any externalization of destructive karma of any man who might be a part of that boatload of individuals entrusted with the mission of carrying the Ascension Flame to Luxor. We had to reach our goal despite any and all individual and collective obstacles, within a given time. How we rejoiced when we reached the mouth of the Nile and knew we were at last within 500 miles of our goal! The tears fell upon our cheeks as, for a moment, we stretched our arms and flexed the muscles in our arms and hands to relieve them from the pressure of service at the oars which we had manned to drive our galley forward when the winds did not fill our sails and help us to reach our goal. We thanked the God that made us as we gazed at the still glowing embers of that Ascension Flame, knowing that within Its presence was the way back Home, not only for ourselves but for all who would lose their bodies in the sinking of Atlantis and who would again wait at the gates of birth for new embodiment upon the remaining landed surface of the Earth. Rising with renewed strength by acknowledgement of our source we rowed up the river to Luxor. I remember the commendable restraint of the members of our company who, rather than rushing over the side of the boat as it rode at anchor, awaited my disembarking, carrying the brazier within which the spark of the Ascension

Flame still burned. Then, forming a dignified procession, all followed me ashore. We knelt about that flame which we had kept alive by our very breath, our prayers and application during the rainy nights at sea, during the foggy days, as the heavy winds beset our slight bark. As we knelt thus, pouring our love into the Ascension Flame, from the embers new Light grew. At the same time, as the great Nile River swelled and the Earth shook, we remembered Atlantis."

The Cataclysm

The cataclysm that occurred 12,000 years ago was accompanied by severe rumblings of the Earth and volcanic explosions. Those erruptions caused the waters to boil. With the exception of five hundred who escaped, the entire population of Poseidonis, sixty million people, lost their lives. The catastrophe lasted less than forty-eight hours.

Besides Poseidonis, other areas were affected as well. During the inferno, the gases locked up in the underground pressure chambers of the Hawaiian Islands were released with such force, that the entire tops of mountains were blown off. The cataclysm formed the islands as they are today. It also caused the draining of the inland sea, which later became part of today's Sahara Desert, and caused the flooding of the Nile.

In the *Mahatma Letters to A.P. Sinnett*, compiled by A. T. Barker (Theosophical Publishing House, Wheaton, Illinois), it is stated in a letter by the Mahatma K.H. (Master Kuthumi), that the remainder of Atlantis, the island of Poseidonis, went down violently, 11,446 years ago. The letter (No. 23B) was written during the year 1882, and according to the editor, all of these letters are stored at the British Museum.

Was the cataclysm that destroyed the Amazon civilization and that severely affected the entire continent of Meru, the same one that destroyed Poseidonis, the last remnant of Atlantis? Some convincing arguments can be given to support this theory.

1) The date for the cataclysm that sank Poseidonis and destroyed Meru (given as 12,000 years ago), was mentioned by the Masters on six different occasions.
2) No other cataclysm of the same or nearly the same extent was given by the Masters as having occurred since that date.
3) The Poseidonis cataclysm affected many parts of the world. Besides submerging Poseidonis, it drained the Sahara inland sea. It also affected, to some extent, areas as far west as Yellowstone Park, and it blew off the tops of the mountains of the Hawaiian Islands. Therefore, it is very likely that it severely affected the nearest coast of Meru, namely its eastern coast.
4) Among all the information given by the Masters, it was never said that any boats leaving Poseidonis arrived on the Eastern coast of Meru. This coast had suffered extensive damage from the cataclysm. The coastline was submerged 160 feet. The Masters knew in advance which part of the world would suffer least from the Poseidonis cataclysm. This can be seen from the fact that some of the priests loyal to Casimir Poseidon were directed to escape to the western part of the United States. They arrived safely since this area received very little damage.
5) The catastrophe lasted an equal amount of time. The Masters stated that the cataclysm that destroyed Poseidonis lasted less than forty-eight hours and the cataclysm that affected Meru

lasted one day.

Some arguments can be made for stating that Noah's flood of Biblical times was caused by the cataclysm 12,000 years ago.

1) When people remember a world-wide cataclysm, the last world-wide cataclysm is foremost in their minds. As time goes on, the memory of earlier cataclysms fades.

   The Masters stated that, unlike the lost continent of Mu, the remembrance of Atlantis and her people has not been entirely forgotten nor obliterated in the history of mankind, but has been recorded in many ways through the centuries, and drifts to us from most unexpected channels.

2) The catastrophe 12,000 years ago must have had a world-wide impact, because:

   a) Not only did Poseidonis sink, but the entire continent of South America felt the effect of the cataclysm.

   b) It caused the explosion of several mountain tops in Hawaii, and caused minor damage at Yellowstone Park.

   c) It drained the inland sea, which area later became part of the Sahara Desert, and it caused the flooding of the Nile.

"Thus, the last remaining fragment of a once world-wide empire sank, to rest for purification, beneath the present Atlantic Ocean. Some of today's myths and legends point to earlier times of glory."

The Masters said that, in time, indisputable proofs both as to Atlantis' existence and its height of attainment, will be revealed by oceanography, geology and other scientific data.

8 - The Time Period From Poseidonis To Jesus

INCAS AND MAYAS

The Meru civilization was followed by a civilization called Pirua, after which the Inca civilization came into existence. All of these civilizations were located in South America. The Incas had a colony in the state of Oaxaca, Mexico. The central focus of this colony was at today's Mitla. A magnificent temple, built partially underground, was located here.

The Pirua and Inca civilizations lasted for thousands of years. What archaeologists have found so far (as of 1930), concerning the Inca civilization, pertains to the state when it was in its decline. The Masters have said that future finds will attest to the great height of that civilization.

The Incas had a skin color similar to that of the American Indian; they were dark-eyed and dark-haired. Unlike the civilizations of Egypt, Atlantis, and the Sahara, those embodied as the masses of the Incan people were not of advanced development. The leaders of the Pirua and Inca civilizations were, however, of an advanced state of development.

The Incas' devotion to God was very great, and

they were taught a good understanding and working knowledge of Cosmic Law and the activity of the Central Sun. The Inca ruler was assisted by Saint Germain. Saint Germain's name at that time was "Son Uriel."

The following information on the Mayan civilization was published in October 1962, fourteen months after Geraldine Innocenti left this plane of existence. Based on the format and substance of the dictation, it appears likely that the dictation was originally given through Ms. Innocenti, and therefore is included in this publication. A summary of this message will now be given.

Many years before the Christian dispensation a Golden Age existed in the province of Yucatan. Under the guidance of its wise ruler, Kenich Ahan (since ascended), the life-giving activity of the Sun, under the direction of Helios and Vesta, was acknowledged and worshipped. Gold was used freely to adorn people and temples, and everyone understood and obeyed God's laws.

Before their conquest by Cortez, Kenich Ahan and the people of the White Priesthood inscribed the entire constructive history of this civilization on fifty-two golden plates. These plates are preserved in a sacred mountain called Uxmal, fifty miles from Merida. "To the ordinary tourist of today it is merely a large mound of earth, containing within and upon its surface the remnants of various temples."

"The lifestreams who originally assisted Kenich Ahan (730 in number) will some day be responsible for making this focus visible to all mankind, showing it to be the most glorious and magnificent ever known."

EGYPT

The action of the Ascension Flame, together with the right use of knowledge and power, brought Egypt to her greatest height. Several large temples were built at Luxor by Ramases II. There were oracles during this time, similar to an action later experienced at Delphi, Greece.

When the oracles began to speak from hidden places, the destruction of Egypt came. Destructive forces had placed some human beings friendly to their cause, acting as oracles, in these places. At a later time this downfall of the civilization was hastened when very advanced lifestreams, who rebelled against the restraint of their lower nature (misuse of sex), embodied. They also were proud of their intellectual accomplishments. Then, also, the priests and priestesses engaged in corrupt practices, creating their own gods to deceive mankind. The Masters said of this activity, "a more corrupt priesthood has never been."

Centuries passed. Egypt entered the dark ages, and the Ascension Temple was located underground and camouflaged for protective purposes. Many of the early Israelites were guests at the temple; Joseph, who was to rise next to the throne of Egypt, Moses, Aaron, Miriam and those who were to be instrumental in the Exodus.

The library of the temple contains books from every civilization that ever existed. The Masters saved some books during the fire that took place at the famous Alexandria Library, and brought them to the Ascension Temple. Other priceless books are guarded by the Brotherhood, and are located in Tibet, China, and other places. They will be brought forth at a time when there is assurance that there will not be a repetition of the fire at Alexandria.

After the Egyptian civilization, other civilizations that followed and achieved great heights were those of Chaldea, Babylonia and Greece.

MOSES

The fifth dispensation started in the year 2,000 B.C., when Moses led the Jewish people from Egypt, where they had suffered. Much of the Mosaic Law was embedded into Moses′ consciousness long before the ascent to the Mount. Moses, Aaron and Miriam had received instructions at the Ascension Temple. Thus is truth conveyed from heart to heart and carried by the feet of many into far places. Moses drew from the Ascension Flame the fire of courage, and Aaron, the arts of the priesthood. No written records were made by priests loyal to the Great White Brotherhood from the time of the sinking of Poseidonis to the time of Moses.

Moses did not gain his ascension in that embodiment. He is now ascended and is known as Lord Ling. He gave some dictations to the students through the messenger Geraldine Innocenti.

LORD GAUTAMA

On May 8, 1958, the Master Lord Gautama gave an extensive dictation about his life. Repeated here is a brief summary of that dictation.

Lord Gautama was born the son of a king in India. He was born without any destructive karma, and was educated in an environment of quiet and beauty. Lovely gardens surrounded the king's palace. The gardens contained the most perfect manifestations of plant and animal life. The servants were requested not to tell the growing boy about imperfect conditions beyond the garden walls.

One day, an event occurred, that changed Lord Gautama's life. He was totally shaken by a careless remark of a servant about conditions of starvation and chaos all over India. Lord Gautama left his father's palace, his wife and baby son, determined to control his energies and to find God-Truth.

He entered a forest and directed his consciousness through the psychic realm surrounding the Earth, finally entering the divine realms of perfection. During this time period of seven years, his physical body remained in the forest. At times Lord Gautama returned in consciousness to the physical realm and partook of food and drink that was left by passing travelers.

Under the loving direction of Pallas Athena and other Ascended Beings, Lord Gautama's consciousness proceeded through the Seven Spheres, the schoolroom of individuals about to enter embodiment upon Earth. He began on the seventh sphere (the sphere most closely located to the Earth), and continued through the other spheres until he reached the first sphere, becoming aware of and absorbing the qualities of each sphere as he went along.

Proceeding still further, he came face to face with the Godhead of our solar system, beloved Helios and Vesta. He saw them, and understood the eternal truth that GOD IS GOOD; that His desire for all His Creation is Good and that the distressing appearances of imperfection upon this Earth WERE NOT GOD'S WILL — NOR ACCORDING TO HIS DIVINE PLAN!

Gradually, Lord Gautama became aware that the enjoyment of the presence of the God-Parents was not enough, and that this enjoyment, also called Nirvana, must yield to the fulfillment of his own divine plan. This meant that Lord Gautama had to bring back his gained knowledge to share on the physical plane with others.

Thus began Lord Gautama's pilgrimage through India. The Hierarchy had hoped that his knowledge of Truth would spread from there to the remainder of the world. During his pilgrimage, Lord Gautama became associated with Ananda (formerly embodied as Moses). However, the mission met with little initial success; just a few monks became believers. Dark forces of the psychic realm would not allow the expansion of the Light to the rest of the world. Through the influence of the Ascended Master Kwan Yin, however, Lord Gautama's teachings were carried to China.

When Lord Gautama's individual divine plan had been fulfilled, He asked the Cosmic Law to be allowed once a year to enter the atmosphere of the Earth in His Ascended Master Body to give his radiation and blessing to the students. The request was granted. This annual occasion is now known as the Wesak Festival.

Lord Gautama explained to the students of the Bridge to Freedom that his original teaching was later distorted. The vow of poverty was not part of his teachings. He said, "This is not God's will! One should not live in foolish poverty, experiencing the lack of any good thing, which, if he had that good to use, would enable him to fulfill his divine plan much more easily, quickly and perfectly."

Lord Gautama taught personal detachment from persons, places, conditions and things — giving no power to illness, distress or any disharmonious external manifestation.

On January 1, 1957, Lord Gautama took Sanat Kumara's place as Lord of the World.

THE GOLDEN AGE OF GREECE

At the same time that Serapis Bey and his group carried the Ascension Flame to the shore of the Nile near Luxor, Hilarion's boat, carrying the Flame of Truth, arrived at Crete. As mentioned before, Crete was connected to Greece at that time.

In previous lives, Hilarion was known as Iamblichus, the neoplatonic writer, and Paul, the Christian Apostle. Inspired by the Flame of Truth, a faithful few embodied again and again. They were assisted by Pallas Athena, Goddess of Truth, and the God Zeus. Together they brought forth the Golden Age of Greece.

The devotees of Truth built a glorious temple on Crete. They used as a blueprint the original Temple of Truth on Poseidonis. After centuries of maintaining a high state of perfection, the Temple of Truth began to fall into decay through the decline of the Grecian civilization. It appears from the dictations that at that time the great palaces of Luxor suffered a similar fate.

The Temple of Truth on Crete was destroyed by those who rebelled against Truth and against the disciplines of purity and harmony. After its destruction, the temple was etherealized; it is still pulsating in the ethers over Crete today.

At a later time, Serapis Bey, in an embodiment as Phidias, rendered a great service to mankind in bringing forth the almost-exact replica of this Temple of Truth. This was done so that the outer consciousness might contemplate its perfection and tune into its service to God. The building was erected near Athens, Greece, about 450 B.C.. It was called the Parthenon, and it was dedicated to Pallas Athena.

Several hundred years before Christ there started in Greece a spiritual order called the Order of Delphi. Most of the individuals associated with this activity had belonged to Pallas Athena's Court. Any Divine Being could use the body of an oracle upon occasion, in order to give instructions to a group who would gather together to receive that assistance. The Masters said that Geraldine Innocenti embodied as an oracle three times.

The first vestal virgins were completely dedicated to magnetizing pure truth. They did draw forth, repeat, and record the truth from beloved Vesta and Pallas Athena. The records still remain within the keeping of the Brotherhood of Truth. Pallas Athena supervised the disciplines and the careful preparations and training necessary for the development of the receptive consciousness of those lifestreams who were to be the mouthpieces of the Brotherhood as the Vestal Virgins of Delphi. They spent their training in solitary confinement, and took the vow to be of pure mind and body. While the priestesses were able to be in tune with the Spirit of truth and listened to the God-voice within, the early Greeks were able to "proceed on the path." This fountain of wisdom was maintained in a state of perfection for almost seven hundred years.

The Masters listed two causes for the decline of the Order of Delphi.

1) Some virgins having much karma were given the opportunity to serve as oracles. They allowed themselves to be bought off by those desiring to forward political causes of their own in the near East, by raising unqualified lifestreams to positions of leadership, thereby making great fortunes. The masses, who had relied upon the Oracles of Delphi for hundreds of years, were now deceived by false prophets. Members of the dark forces wrote out messages and gave them to the oracles, who would deliver

these messages to the unsuspecting people.

2) One Vestal Virgin did not live up to the vow of purity. Contagion spread through the entire order of Delphic Oracles, and brought the order to ruin. This destroyed the connection and contact between beloved Vesta, Pallas Athena, and the people of the Earth.

The people listening to the oracles had come in faith and hope, and it took some time before they realized they had been deceived. Some became so disillusioned that it caused a deep imprint on their etheric bodies, and in later embodiments they remained very suspicious of anything that had to do with mystic phenomena or extra-sensory perception. The Master Hilarion personally devoted a portion of His life to those disappointed lifestreams, hoping to bring them back to the point where they again desire the truth which will set them free.

9 - The Life Of Jesus and Mary

INTRODUCTION

As stated in the foreword, the only source of reference for the text of this part of the book are the dictations of the Ascended Masters as given to the two messengers. These accounts may agree with the Bible and they may not.

Since the emphasis of this publication is on history rather than on Cosmic Law, only a few details of Jesus′ message are repeated here, but it should be emphasized that His teachings correspond in all respects with that of the other Ascended Masters.

Additional information on Jesus′ teachings may be found in the book *Life and Teaching of Jesus and Mary*, by A.D.K. Luk.

THE CHRISTIAN DISPENSATION

Every hundred years, within the 2,000 year cycle, the Lords of Karma give a dispensation of energy to the Spiritual Hierarchy of the Earth. The Lord of the World, the World Teacher, and the Maha Chohan, in council, decide how best to invest that energy. They look upon spiritually-advanced individuals, who may play a role in carrying out the dispensation, they look upon conditions upon the Earth, and they investigate the application of Cosmic Law upon the dispensation. Based on these factors, they present a plan to the entire Great White Brotherhood. Each member then calls upon several chelas, offering them opportunity to participate in the plan, provided they qualify and volunteer for this service.

The Christian Dispensation was worked out at inner levels long before Jesus assumed his mission. The predominant cycle was the sixth ray of devotion, and the dispensation was designed to give the greatest blessing to the lifestreams who would embody during the following 2,000 years, under the beneficial radiation of that ray.

Before individual commitments were made, the entire Christian Dispensation was played upon the Cosmic Screen, showing how it would be first originated and developed by a humble group of individuals; then how the dispensation would mature to a greater intensity as more people would dedicate themselves to such service.

At the close of this presentation, the call was made for volunteers. Jesus, Mary, Joseph, John the Baptist, and the persons who would be Jesus' disciples, were among the people who volunteered and eventually qualified.

Lord Maitreya was required to test the strength of each volunteer, and through the process of initiation some lifestreams were eliminated.

Mary also had to pass a test, which lasted for three hours. During that time Mary had to prove she could hold her attention and hold the concentrated image of Jesus' divine nature as a child of God against any conceivable mental force and pressure directed by a Master at her. At the end of that initiation Mary was given the right to embody and await the coming of Jesus. One reason Mary qualified is that she had been trained in the power of concentration — holding on to one concept at a time — by abiding in temples for elementals during prior ages. She was warned that the test she passed was a small one compared to the one she would be required to pass when the viciousness of some dark forces would be hurled against her. Before Mary took embodiment she did ask for, and was granted a favor that turned out to be most essential to the success of Jesus' mission. She asked Archangel Gabriel to announce to her Jesus' coming, at that time in the future when she would be embodied, and would not retain the consciousness of her mission.

MARY'S CHILDHOOD

As a child, Mary's interests were different from those of the other young girls of Judea. While other children played with dolls, she contemplated all the prophecies of the Old Testament, and developed a great devotion to the Beloved Vesta. (Helios and Vesta govern our Solar system.) She drew from Vesta the feeling of divine mother-love.

At the age of three Mary was taken by her parents,

Joachim and Anne, to the Temple at Luxor for instruction. There she remained until she attained maturity. It was a lonely life for a small child, and the severe disciplines were not softened even for one so young. The priests trained her in the powers of concentration. In this way she would be prepared for her later mission, to hold unwaveringly the "immaculate concept," which is the divine concept of man, for her child, Jesus. While her young friends enjoyed children's games and played in the grasses, Mary, at the age of five, was given the chore of copying letters from the scriptures. Her task was to keep her attention on her work, and to not be distracted by the shining sun or the sound of the children at play. During her stay at the temple Mary had to pass some severe tests and initiations. She stated to the students that she hoped no unascended being would ever have to go through such tests again.

In the afternoon Mary would find rest and solitude by going to a quiet place where she would have the comfort of her twin-flame, Archangel Raphael. She enjoyed very much the happiness of that association, and the beauty of that companionship.

Mary grew in beauty and grace, and the angels were a constant companion, enjoying the beauty of her company. There was practically no veil between the angelic kingdom and her own sweet self. She was truly a "Queen of the Angels."

Later on, just before her release from the temple, the remembrance of her association with the angels grew more dim. During that time Mary had to ponder in her heart the oneness of God and His perfect creation, man. Mary explained to the students that the type of comradeship and friendship between the individual and his God-Presence, established in everyday tasks of life, builds a momentum for him. She continued, stating that she never set a table, never swept a floor, never planted a flower, without doing so with the realization that it was the life of God that enabled her to do this task, and she performed it for the glory of God. Mary's entire youth was dedicated to preparing for the hour when her mission would begin in earnest.

After her release from the temple, Mary was awaiting the appearance of her guardian. Her first meeting with Joseph was a memorable one, because above Joseph (now the Ascended Master Saint Germain) she saw the blazing figure of Archangel Zadkiel. To Mary that was the confirmation that Joseph was the proper and chosen guardian for her.

Joseph was a member of the Essene Brotherhood, and a very advanced, spiritual man. He had a very good knowledge of Cosmic Law, and he imparted that knowledge to Mary. It was his quiet strength, his serenity, and dignity that helped Mary during many of the difficult experiences later in her life.

JESUS' CHILDHOOD AND HIS TRAINING

From the day Mary was taken to the temple for her training, she lived in a state of constant "listening grace." So it was easy for Archangel Gabriel to fulfill the pledge he had given to Mary before her embodiment, approaching her with the triumphant words, "Hail, Mary, full of grace." He conveyed to Mary that through her body would come the physical form of Jesus, who would be the Messiah. It was required of Mary to tell this event to no one but Joseph. If Mary had not been in a constant state of listening grace, which means to be always prepared to listen to the still small voice within, she would have missed Gabriel's message.

Mary and Joseph prepared for the birth of Jesus.

Mary made small garments for the infant, and together they planned their future so they might have the strength to fulfill their mission in glory.

Jesus was born at a time when the collective constructively-qualified energy of the Earth was at its lowest level since the days of Atlantis. His coming and successful mission turned the tide.

Jesus was born without karma. According to a dictation given by Jesus in 1953, in previous embodiments he was Appollonius of Tyana, Zoroaster in Persia, and Joshua.

The now Ascended Master El Morya (who was one of the "Three Wise Men," together with the now Ascended Masters Kuthumi and Djwal Kul) recalls his former embodiment as follows:

> "I, too, followed a Star once long ago, to the feet of an infant. I can assure you it was not as glamorous or romantic or beautiful as it is described today, and that the Three Kings of the Orient did not ride easily in great caravans of power and wealth. We joined them, it is true, for travelers in those days seldom crossed those vast expanses of waste land alone, but we were within garments of flesh. We had studied the heavens for many years, each in his own country. We had no communication one with the other and each, when the constellations pointed to the certain Cosmic moment, felt the time of a Visitation was at hand, and each, at some sacrifice, suffering, and much ridicule from our countrymen, left the comparative safety of our homes, following a star. There were nights when the clouds covered the heavens and the stars did not shine — just as there are times in your progress upon the spiritual path when your star seems to be obliterated from the sky, and even in your feelings you wonder if there ever is such a 'guiding Light.'"
>
> "I can understand this because I went every step of that way, following a star, and I can assure you,

with the confidence and faith built into my own energies, that it was worth the investment of every electron drawn forth from the heart of the Presence, and used in motivating the body toward that humble stall in Bethlehem."

Jesus said in 1953 that the now Ascended Masters El Morya and Kuthumi, and those engaged in the study of the stars, knew that the hour for his conception and embodiment was about to take place.

Jesus' mission had to comply with the laws as they applied to the Earth at that time. He did not receive special privileges, such as the gift of consecutive consciousness. He was bound by the "bands of forgetfulness" like any other lifestream seeking his evolution upon the planet Earth. Therefore, when he awoke as a beautiful baby in Mary's arms, or later, when he grew older, he did not remember any former embodiments. (A.D.K. Luk reports that Jesus, as part of his mission, did receive the privilege of being able to transmute an additional amount of karma. Therefore he was able to bring about more healings than he would have been able to without such a privilege.)

It was well that a great momentum had been established between Mary and the angelic kingdom, because shortly after the birth of Jesus an angel brought news of impending disaster.

One night soon after the birth of Jesus, Mary saw Joseph standing in the doorway. He was deeply troubled. Joseph said that he had just received a warning. He was not sure of the source. Was it an angel and was it of God? The impression on his consciousness was to flee at once and go to Egypt. Joseph had misgivings. He felt it was unfair for a newborn child, having such a mission, to so soon be the subject of the cruelty of Herod. Together they prayed, and Mary received confirmation in her heart that they should go. As behind them the blood of the infants flowed in the streets, Mary (and Jesus later on) vowed then she would personally assist each child that was involved in such an act of brutality, to gain the ascension in a future embodiment. These children had died because of their mission. Mary took her small baby, and together with Joseph, left the shelter of their home and journeyed to Egypt, a land filled with dangerous wildlife. It was a long, tedious ride into Egypt, with many sleepless nights, fleeing before Herod's soldiers.

When Jesus was a very small boy, he already manifested a purity of spirit. His senses were also well developed. He had perfect sight, perfect hearing, perfect taste, touch and smell. Besides this, he had great intuition.

Jesus did not live in a "privileged, charmed world." He lived in the midst of so-called imperfection. He was called upon to rub shoulders with the poor, and the sick of mind and body. There were no public institutions at that time to take such individuals away from public life. The beautiful boy, dressed in his simple white tunic and the sandals that Joseph had made for him, was exposed to the pressures of thoughts from many planes, with only the love of Mary and Joseph protecting him.

Jesus' parents were his earliest teachers. Mary told him that it was entirely up to him, to either accept the world filled with imperfections, such as the appearance of illness and distress, as real, or to "magnify the Lord." Jesus later stated to the students that this lesson helped him immensely in his later mission and "preserved his sanity many times." Joseph also often applied this principle.

Mary stated there is always that choice — to either tune in to and magnify the appearance world, or to choose to magnify the power of God, by turning the beam of one's energy and attention to one's I AM Presence, holding one's attention focused there until the inner self gains in confidence. When young Jesus came to Mary with bruises on his feet and knees she would say: "We shall not magnify the hurt or that scar. We shall magnify our Lord." Then, turning her attention to the perfect pattern, the man made in God's image and likeness, Mary, Joseph and Jesus would draw the healing and peace currents of their God-Presence through them, until the appearance of imperfection would disappear. This they did systematically, every day. Thus, together they built a momentum that was to be the foundation for meeting the difficult days ahead; yes, for overcoming death itself.

When Mary and Joseph were in Egypt they had many experiences which tested their faith and power of concentration. One morning Mary saw young Jesus playing on the shore of the Nile River. Suddenly a large crocodile appeared next to him. The crocodile had its mouth open. For a moment, Mary was stunned. Then she gathered her senses, visualizing Jesus enfolded in God's protection until the crocodile finally swam away. Jesus did not think there was anything unusual about this experience, he just waved to his mother and went on playing.

At the tender age of five, Jesus entered the temple of Luxor and, as it was with Mary, the severe discipline of the priests of the temple was re-experienced. Mary was not permitted to witness his training. She had to wait outside the temple in the hot sun, shaded by a fig tree, while young Jesus received instructions from early morning until well into the afternoon. Sometimes, after leaving the temple, Mary noticed beads of perspiration on his forehead, and deep circles under his eyes. He had to undergo tests and disciplines from which fullgrown men and women have shrunk, yet Mary could not interfere. It was her obligation to give him complete freedom, a freedom within which there is no fear.

Of his childhood, Jesus said in 1961: "I too, awoke

to a world of form, to a world of shadows, and had to find within myself the reason and purpose of my being. Well do I remember those early days in Egypt when I was taken at a tender age into those temples, when I learned the Law before the priests. I do recall my gratitude for the love of my mother and father, which balanced the austerity, the discipline, the tremendous pressure required of even a child, who applied for mastery in one of the temples at Luxor."

While Mary was not permitted to accompany Jesus to the temple, she was privately given the same lessons by the Hierarch of the temple, Serapis Bey. That instruction was on the suspension of the breath, and the resurrection of the body, thus preparing her for events to come.

When Jesus reached maturity, with the assistance of Joseph, he became a skilled carpenter. Later on, Joseph made many important contributions in establishing the Christian Era. He first introduced Jesus to the disciples.

Joseph knew of those disciples for years before Jesus was aware of them. He contacted those men by explaining to them how his study of ancient prophecies and teachings of the Law showed that the Messiah would come soon, but that it was up to each one to recognize the Messiah for himself. In other words, Joseph did not tell them that Jesus was the Messiah. Rather, they had to discern the reality of the Messiah for themselves through the feelings from within their own hearts when they met him. Later, Joseph taught the disciples as much as their individual consciousnesses would absorb, and as much as the Law would permit at that time.

James and John the Beloved were orphans. They were raised by a kind woman, and Joseph was their guardian. As the woman was getting along in age, Joseph asked the two boys which one would accept the responsibility as head of the household, and which one would be willing to be trained by the Essene Brotherhood. As it turned out, James, the older and more practical one, took the responsibilities of the household, and John went to the Essenes for many years of training. This way he would be prepared to be the "right-hand" of Jesus. James subsequently went to Galilee, where he met Peter and Andrew.

Luke was a physician who had received some private instructions from Jesus in healing. He was not totally convinced of Jesus' healing powers and other accomplishments, and would often say: "I do not believe it can be done."

During Jesus' growing years it was Joseph's service to be his teacher. When Jesus' contact with the Ascended Master Lord Maitreya was developed to the point that there was practically no veil between them anymore, Lord Maitreya became his new teacher.

One day Joseph told Mary that his mission in life was nearly accomplished. He asked her to stay in Bethany after he left this plane. There she would be in the hands of friends. Jesus, he said, was to go to India to receive some important message. Shortly thereafter, Joseph passed from this scene of life.

Joseph had not been gone very long when Jesus found himself going alone, on foot, to India in a simple, solitary pilgrimage. He entered India, following the vague directions of Joseph, having to depend on the dictates of his own I AM Presence. He came upon a group of people seated around a teacher, and sat silently with them. The teacher's name was "Great Divine Director," an Ascended Master. The Master did not acknowledge his arrival, but mentally projected to him the words "I AM the Resurrection and the Life" and "I AM the Ascension in the Light." That was the entire contact between Jesus and the teacher. Jesus got up and walked back home, grateful that he had received the key words for his mission.

After Jesus returned from Egypt, prior to his public

ministry, he and Mary went back to Luxor, Egypt, once more. Here they stayed for three years. Both of them mastered the final initiation of the Luxor Retreat, which is the conscious removal of the life currents from the body, and the returning of them through the controlled breath. This was done to prepare them for Jesus' supreme test. Twelve Masters stood watch over their bodies during that period, and both Jesus and Mary passed the test victoriously.

A.D.K. Luk states: "Jesus, from the age of twelve to twenty-eight received training in various retreats and monasteries, among them a monastery in the Kashmir Valley, where he stayed for five years. There are scrolls preserved here which Jesus wrote himself."

THREE MAGNIFICENT YEARS

Jesus' mission started at the age of thirty. His ministry lasted three years. This three-year time limit was predetermined by Cosmic Law. He spoke in simple terms and in easy-to-understand parables, so that the man on the street could understand. From a spiritual viewpoint, Jesus touched less than 500 life-streams. This was partially due to the difficult conditions of travel prevailing at that time.

During the time Jesus was engaged in his mission, Mary stayed with Martha and the "other Mary" (possibly Mary of Bethany), on the outskirts of Bethany. Here there was an old mill that had been used to grind corn. There was a certain peacefulness in the simplicity of country living. Mary enjoyed this environment and wove garments for Jesus. Once a day she walked up the small and grassy mound to a great flat-topped rock. There she spent several hours in deep and earnest communion with God. In this manner she built the momentum and the pattern upon which Jesus and Mary later ascended. When Jesus rested between trips, he visited Mary at Bethany, and in those moments both found happiness during this difficult time.

Jesus' first so-called miracle was the changing of water to "wine" at the wedding in Cana. He turned his attention to God, and through the energies of his spiritual momentum, changed the substance of that water into electronic light. It was the people who unconsciously qualified it with what they desired to manifest. Therefore, the substance they drank tasted to them like wine.

The "feeding of the five thousand" was accomplished using similar principles. Jesus multiplied the loaves and the fish using the Law of Precipitation. The bread and fish were multiplied by drawing together electronic light-substance, the substance which is around us in the atmosphere. This substance was drawn into form, and then lowered into a lower vibratory action, enabling the people to eat what looked and tasted like fish. (As recorded in the book, *Unveiled Mysteries*, Saint Germain used the same concepts of Law in giving Mr. Ballard a milky liquid which was also produced from electronic light substance. This greatly refreshed and revitalized Mr. Ballard.)

From early childhood on, Jesus was taught to magnetize PEACE. That peace became a great reservoir. It enabled Jesus to say with authority, "Peace, be still." The turbulent waters of the sea of Galilee responded. This feeling of peace was also present, when He said, "Love your enemies, treat kindly those who despitefully use you."

Invoking all the gathered momentum of LIFE EVERLASTING, and directing that energy into the heart of Lazarus, Jesus was able to render a service. The energy he called forth was more powerful than the moaning, crying, curiosity, skepticism and other qualities of an imperfect nature acting through the people who were present. Lazarus responded, and came forth from the so-called dead.

While performing his many miracles, Jesus had the spiritual assistance of Almighty God, his teacher Lord Maitreya, and his mother, Mary. Jesus, in a dictation, urged the students to be prepared at all times to use their God-given abilities. One never knows when this opportunity comes. He said: "The moment is NOW! Do not consult the calendar as to when to do a certain thing! I was not told beforehand what to experience. I had no written scroll, saying on such and such a date the Holy Spirit would descend, and on such and such a date I was to heal."

Jesus stated in a dictation to the students in 1961, "Through misinterpretation of the Law I was unfortunately set apart as the "Only Begotten Son." I came to bring the example of eternal life, overcoming, through the assistance of Divine Beings, the experience called death. Then I had to convince my disciples that I still lived and moved among them, resurrected. All of these things I did because the world required then, and now, the coming of a perfect one, one who can fulfill the purpose, and represent on Earth, one Heavenly Father. Have you ever been whipped in public, with a crown of thorns pressed into your brow? Have you had your garments rent? No! The things which have happened to you during this embodiment are very slight compared to those experiences through which I voluntarily passed to show that the Son of God was the master of energy in this world."

In 1961, beloved Mary said, "The diabolical forces still roam through the world, emphasizing the wrong part of Jesus′ mission. They glorify a crucified Christ, muting a resurrected Christ." Jesus′ words add emphasis as follows: "The crucified Christ, which the orthodox world places before the people, is the symbol of vicarious atonement. It is the way of the outer self to let some other lifestream carry your sin. THE CRUCIFIED CHRIST IS TO BE REPLACED BY THE ASCENDED CHRIST." It is up to each individual to atone for his own sins.

Addressing himself to the present accuracy and authenticity of the Bible, the Maha Chohan explained in 1960 that there were some Bible scholars who embellished upon the original text. (No wonder we have over 100 different "Christian Faiths!")

In his dictations Jesus again and again stressed that the miracles of 2,000 years ago can again be accomplished TODAY by the students. He also mentioned that only since the 1927 dispensation, has the apex of that service been reached which he expects to render. As part of this service OPPORTUNITY is given to the students of Ascended Masters as seldom before in the history of the earth. "These students," He said, "alone are the hope of the Earth. Churches have had their opportunities for 2,000 years to set mankind free, yet the people have grown into greater and greater bondage. I implore you, in the name of the Father of all life, IF YOU LOVE ME, DO THAT WHICH I HAVE DONE!"

THE CRUXIFIXION

After the disciples and the Master had finished the "Last Supper," and had gone to Gethsemane, Mary, another lady whose name was also Mary, and Martha gathered together the linen cloth which Mary had woven, and folded it carefully. Mary knew deep within herself that within one day that cloth would enfold the body of her yet vital, beautiful son. The cup of the last supper was wrapped in a napkin and given to Joseph of Arimathea for safe-keeping. Then Mary engaged in earnest prayer, for the next day was to bring the greatest trial of her life.

Several times before, Jesus and Mary had discussed the various points that were to be emphasized during his ministry. Often they talked over the necessity of passing through the appearance of death in order to prove the immortality of life.

At Luxor it was comparatively easy for the highly-trained initiate to withdraw the senses from contact with the world around him and suspend the breath, so that, to the outer sense the body was "dead." However, to perform this act consciously, amid hundreds of vicious consciousnesses, is much more difficult. Yet, in order to satisfy the outer consciousness, it was necessary for mankind itself to actually perform and execute the death sentence. Otherwise, mankind would never have believed that the resurrection was authentic, and that it was not a trick of a fakir or a manifestation of hypnosis.

Mary said that neither she nor Jesus relished the necessity of having to pass through this experience. When Jesus asked that the "cup" be taken from him, it was because no one knew for certain whether or not the public demonstration would be successful. Through such a public experience, all of the astral and psychic viciousness that had accumulated since the "fall of man" was directed through those embodied individuals who allowed themselves to be used as pawns or shells of that force.

Standing in the wind on Calvary's hilltop, looking at the greed in the consciousness of those who loved and enjoyed the spectacle, Mary, with every fibre and cell of her being, held to the perfect concept of the resurrected, risen, breathing Christ. She called to Lord Maitreya, to Helios and Vesta, to Gabriel and to everyone who had given her assistance before. Mary sensed the response from the heart of the Sun; she saw the Presence of Vesta; she saw above Jesus the luminous, shining Presence of Lord Maitreya, and the nearness of Gabriel.

Mary also remembered Joseph. She missed his serene, physical presence. She thought of a winter night long ago, and of a simple stable. [This statement suggests that the Biblical account of the time and location of the birth of Jesus is correct.] Mary remembered the long, tedious ride to Egypt, and the entrance to the temple. She thought of the disciples not yet anchored in the understanding of what was really happening. All those thoughts came to her, and yet Mary was able to hold her attention upon what she called the "immaculate concept" of Jesus, knowing that neither the spear nor the crown of thorns, nor the cross, nor the nails could hurt him. As it turned out, a series of humble, daily experiences, into which all the energies of Mary's bodies were poured, built a form which proved to be her strength, balance and sanity in the hour of need. She stood and upheld the focus of the Resurrection Flame upon her son, and concentrated her energies upon the victorious, happy pattern of her life experiences.

As always, Mary was able to see Jesus' Holy Christ Self (the Master explained elsewhere that the Christ Self abides above the physical vehicle).

For three long hours Jesus' body hung between that of two thieves on the cross.

John assisted Mary, holding to that Perfect Concept of man as co-creator with God, so that Jesus might pass through that initiation, resuscitating his physical form, resurrecting it on Easter Morning for the benefaction of a doubting discipleship, and finally, ascending in the sight of over 500 people.

According to A.D.K. Luk, Mary and John understood how to disconnect, through Light and love, the gravity pull of the physical body. This they applied as the cross was raised, thus preventing the tearing of his body. Continuing with this account, Jesus' last words were not "My God, My God, why hast thou forsaken me?" but, "Father, how thou hast glorified me; into Thy hands I command my Spirit." Then the words "It is finished," were heard coming from the direction of the cross.

Jesus did experience pain from the physical abuse inflicted upon him prior to the crucifixion. But he did not suffer while being on the cross, because he was master of the situation, and had withdrawn from the body sufficiently so that he did not feel pain. Unfortunately, some churches focus upon the agony and distress of Jesus while being on the cross.

At the birth of Jesus the "Three Wise Men" gave him frankincense and myrrh. These items had been kept carefully by Mary, and were used by Martha and the "other Mary" in annointing the body of Jesus, and wrapping it in the linen furnished by Mary. The body was now ready for entombment.

THE RESURRECTION

John and Mary left it to the others to perform the final rites. Accompanied by a feeling of inner peace, they walked down Calvary Hill in the direction of Bethany. They stayed at the old mill, located on the outskirts of the town. Here they found refuge and solace from the pressures of the past events.

Mary asked to be left alone, and for two nights and one day she concentrated on the action of the Resurrection Flame, assisting in restoring the broken body of Jesus. She prayed for many hours, finally falling asleep at her vigil. Then through her mind came the magnificent, melodious voice of Gabriel. He entered her consciousness, using the same words he used when he confirmed Jesus' messiahship, namely, "Hail, Mary! Full of grace!"

At first Mary thought she was dreaming of the earlier visitation. But Gabriel confirmed, "Your son is risen! He is victorious! The tomb has been shattered. He inhabits his body and I come — the Announcer — the Protector of the 'Immaculate Concept' — to bring you the first word of victory!"

Mary fell to her knees, acknowledging Gabriel's presence, and tears of gratitude streamed down her face. The room was filled with light, and scented with the fragrance of the lily. As the brilliant light softened, Mary could recognize Jesus, clothed in the same white robe that she had woven for him. She was even able to recognize her own stitching in the hem of his garment. As she examined his features to be sure it was not a mirage, Jesus reached out his hands and spoke to her saying, "Mother, it is I!"

Mary rushed toward him, touching his robe, thinking to kiss the hem, but he raised her up. Together they walked to the window to look at the sun, which, as a symbol of Life and Light they had worshipped and loved as an outer manifestation of God.

When Mary looked at Jesus' hands, she noticed there were still scar marks caused by the nails; the marks on the forehead from the thorns were gone, however. Jesus explained that an Ascended Being had suggested to him to keep the marks on the hands and feet, as well as the spear mark, as a means of identification.

Jesus parted from her, explaining he had to see Martha, Mary of Magdelene, Peter, James, and John because they were totally shaken by the crucifixion, and much afraid. Before leaving, Jesus asked Mary if she wished to ascend with him, or whether she wanted to stay on (Mary apparently had qualified for the ascension, as had Jesus). Mary countered his question, asking what he wanted her to do. Jesus answered, explaining that it would take an unascended being to magnetize and anchor the cosmic currents for the Christian Dispensation. Mary happily agreed to stay, which pleased him. Now Jesus told Mary he had received a special new dispensation (from the Karmic Board) under which it was possible for him to visit with her and John for thirty years, to give them certain points of Law that here-to-fore were not allowed to be given. As part of the plan to anchor the currents, it was required that at all times either John or Mary were to stay in Bethany.

Jesus added that he was also permitted to visit with Mary and others for forty days prior to his ascension, to explain the Law to them. He said he would send Peter, James, Andrew, John, Luke and the women who loved them, to Bethany.

When Jesus contacted his disciples after the resurrection, he was no longer operating in his physical body, he was operating in his Christ Self. While in the tomb, in cooperation with the Maha Chohan and Archangel Gabriel, Jesus had transmuted his physical body by sending light rays from his I AM Presence, drawing the purified essence of the physical body into the Christ-Self.

Jesus was then functioning in his pure light body, in which every atom and electron was under Jesus' conscious control. Therefore, he could vary the vibratory action of the Christ-Self at will, enabling him to make it visible and tangible to the degree he wished. This light body required no food or drink, and had no flesh or bones, but Jesus could make it appear to look like a flesh body to the disciples to convince them of his tangible presence. Raising the vibratory action of his Christ-Self body, he could go through walls of buildings without difficulty. Having gained mastery over matter (energy, substance and vibration), he could even assist the disciples in doing physical work.

Why did Jesus not simply ascend from the cross?

Mary explained that Jesus could have done so, but the action of the Resurrection Flame was chosen, to strengthen the faith of the disciples, and to establish a focus for the Christian Era.

By appearing each day to Mary and the disciples, sometimes for minutes, sometimes for hours, for forty days, their feelings became anchored in the supremacy of the laws of Almighty God. The disciples had to learn that it is possible for EVERY student of truth to apply the law and have the victory of its manifestation. Mary said in a dictation, "WHAT ONE HAS DONE, ALL MAY ONE DAY DO."

The establishment of a focus which would live for 2,000 years on the Light (constructive, qualified energy) of Jesus and Mary, and which would have the vitality, the fire, and the necessary strength to sustain itself when both had ascended, was necessary to the Christian Dispensation.

It was decided to remodel the living quarters of the old mill, as it was sort of run down. Also, since it was being used as an assembly room for Jesus' visits, it had to accommodate more people. First, a small room was provided for Mary, inside the mill. Then Jesus suggested digging a ditch to irrigate Mary's garden, to save her steps in carrying water. A stream of water flowed behind the mill, adding to the peace and beauty of the scenery. Mary was interested in herbs, which she had planted for their healing power. So the old mill became the focus of the Christian Dispensation, and Mary stayed here for another 30 years.

Jesus not only gave advice, but he also helped with the work of renovating. At one time he helped strengthen a roof beam by adding a support column. In this way the span of the beam would be shortened. Peter cut a tree; Jesus, using his carpenter skills, planed it down, and together they placed the support column in the center of the room. James, John, and

Peter white-washed the living quarters.

As said before, when Jesus was giving instruction or was helping with the renovating, he was operating in the body of his Christ Self, not yet in the Ascended Master body of his I AM Presence.

Gifts came from many places. Joseph of Arimathea sent some sheep. These provided the wool for the garments. Pilate's wife, a lovely person, contributed some imported milking-goats. In a letter she asked permission to visit. The friends of Judas Iscariot and his family offered forty fig and olive trees. These were gratefully accepted and planted.

In the evenings the small community gathered, and Mary told them about Jesus' birth and his life. Matthew, Mark and John wrote the story using their own words. Sometimes Mary made corrections. In this way the Gospels were written.

Finally, the end of the forty-day-period approached. This time the parting was much easier and happier. Everyone had a much better understanding of the Law, and knew within their hearts that the Christ would be with them always, even if the physical form of Jesus would not be present any longer.

Jesus promised John that he would receive his ascension at the close of his embodiment. He had earned it through his love and fidelity to the cause, and because of his service and care of Mary. Mary said later to the students: "On every occasion when I required help, John always stood by. Truly, he was love."

THE ASCENSION

While Mary was staying at Bethany, she walked up the hill alone each day, weaving a pattern of light. While on her way, she prayed and sent her love and gratitude to God, sending forth her invocations for Jesus′ victory. This pathway of Light pierced through the physic realm, connecting with the consciousness of Vesta. Over this pathway Jesus later would walk in his triumph. The rising of energy from her heart built the pattern of the Ascension Flame, used to gain Jesus′ victory.

A dispensation which governs an entire race at the changing of a 2,000-year cycle is composed of the combined, woven energies of many concentrated life-streams. This was the case at the beginning of the Christian Dispensation, and such was the case when, during the 1930′s and 1950′s the Ascended Masters Saint Germain and El Morya drew forth the lifestreams to constructively qualify energy in group activities to anchor the 2,000-year cycle of the New Age.

The night before the ascension, Jesus spoke to Mary and John. He explained that he would climb the hill of Bethany alone early in the morning. Mary, John, and the disciples were to hold the crowd back until about nine o′clock. Then they all could follow him.

The morning came, and Jesus walked up the hill alone. His presence acted like a magnet. His aura was just as it was before, when he was on his mission, so magnetic and powerful, that even when people were asleep, they arose and followed him.

Mary instructed the disciples to hold the crowd back, just as Jesus had asked. In order to keep the people harmonious, Mary told the multitude stories of

Jesus' life.

At 9 o'clock the crowd followed Jesus up the hill. His garments were already brilliant, and people noticed his radiance reflected in the atmosphere. So bright was the light shining through his body, that Mary and the others could scarcely look upon it. He spoke no more. Mary and the disciples prayed for him, holding their concentration on the Ascension Flame. Then from the top of the hill, from the very rock upon which Mary had spent countless hours in prayer, Jesus ascended into the electronic body of his I AM Presence. This was witnessed by five hundred people.

In a dictation to the students in the 1950's, Jesus gave the account of his ascension as follows:

"John and Mother Mary chose to guard that place for me, and thus on that morning, I was enabled to quietly and unostentatiously walk up that grassy path to the top of Bethany's Hill, and have just a little solitude, watching the sun rise, enjoying the beauties of Earth before my beloved disciples and those who came to wonder and to question, reached the brow of the hill. So it was, in that resurrected body, that I was able, in the presence of almost five hundred people, not all of whom believed that such a thing was possible, to quicken the vibratory action of that resurrected form, and with the great assistance of the mighty prayer force that my mother had established through her years of prayer on Bethany's Hill, together with the great assistance of my own I AM Presence, the ascension was publicly manifest.

"Some there were who saw it, some there were who did not, because as the light became brighter, the natural activity of the human self was to cover the eyes against glare. Some were frightened, and turned their backs lest they be distressed. Some flung themselves to the ground, but the few who stood could bear witness. I ascended to my Father and to yours, enjoying that company of Divine Beings who have foresworn

Nirvana, continuing my assistance as best I could to any and all lifestreams, who in their turn would direct their attention toward me."

In a dictation in the 1950's, Jesus said to the students that when he walked up the hill at Bethany, there was still a choice to remain on Earth. He also said that the hardest thing of his life was to leave Mary and the others behind.

According to the account given by Jesus and Mary, Jesus was wearing the robe that Mary had furnished him, when he ascended. The robe and the body of the Christ Self were etherealized when Jesus stepped into the electronic body of his I AM Presence. This was done according to Cosmic Law, which states that anything that has fulfilled its usefulness should be committed to the Flame to be etherealized, returning to original substance. [Therefore, it appears that the "Shroud of Turin" (the linen that Jesus's body was wrapped in) is not authentic. Also, when comparing the imprint of the head of the shroud with a painting of Jesus which I regard as genuine, I find a different proportion of the dimensions of his head.]

PENTECOST

After the crucifixion and resurrection, the Roman government and the Sanhedrin (High Priests) were content and satisfied. They felt certain they had put an end to this menace to their authority. As far as they were concerned, things were now nice and quiet.

Jesus suggested to his friends to keep it that way, and to not draw undue attention to their small community in Bethany. He asked that an upper room in Jerusalem be rented where the disciples and Mary could meet. Matthew was the keeper of the funds, and so it was his responsibility to secure a room. The purpose of the meeting was to restore the disciples' confidence and faith, which was fading somewhat after Jesus' ascension.

Those who knew of the coming of the Holy Spirit prepared for the first Pentecost. The meaning of 'Holy Spirit' has confounded many. Simply put, it is the life-giving, life-supporting energy (prana) radiated from the Central Sun, and directed to the Earth. Here it is received and further projected by the Maha Chohan (Lord of Rays). Therefore, the Maha Chohan is not the Holy Spirit, as He is commonly called, but rather, he DIRECTS the Holy Spirit. The triune action of "Father, Son, and the Holy Spirit" is nothing more that God, His Creation (the Son), and the Life-giving energy radiated by the Central Sun (Holy Spirit). Simple is the Law of Life.

The first Pentecost consisted of an additional amount of prana released to the assembly. It had a profound effect upon the disciples. When the radiation of the Holy Spirit occurred, the disciples were filled anew with vital fire. In fact, they were filled with so much energy that they appeared drunken to others. It gave new emphasis to their lives; it was the final act in preparing them to meet the public to preach the Gospel.

Mary was greatly relieved, because during those ten days after the ascension, many had leaned on her for faith and confidence, and she was mentally exhausted. Now, after Pentecost, the disciples became much more self-reliant.

THE JOURNEY TO GREAT BRITAIN

After Pentecost, the small community at Bethany enjoyed comparative peace for a time. The disciples taught the law to those who wanted to know. From the wool of the sheep the women wove the garments. Together they planted grain, flax and trees. In the evening the Gospels were written. Peter, John, and James wrote Gospels that remain hidden to this day. Mary also wrote some treatises on mystical healing that have never been publicized. Concerning the latter, Mary said in the 1950's that she hoped to bring them to the students at a later date.

One day, a message was received by Joseph of Arimathea, who had extensive business holdings on the British Isles. He had to leave for this destination, and extended an invitation to Mary and the disciples to accompany him.

Jesus had told Mary previously that it would be necessary before her ascension to carry the "Cup" to the British Isles. It was felt that now the opportunity had presented itself to accomplish that purpose. In addition, it was learned that Pilate had been replaced by the Roman government, and the new governor was known to be less lenient toward the Christians than Pilate had been. Therefore, it was considered wise to have Mary leave Bethany for some time.

Joseph of Arimathea had many slaves to man his boat. Mary reminded him that a mission involving the carrying of the sacred Cup to Britain could not involve slave labor. Joseph agreed, and the boats were manned by volunteers from the Christian community. The boats had sails and oars. By volunteering and carrying out their mission as oarsmen, these men won the privilege of being the first knights of King Arthur's Court in a later embodiment.

John was left behind. Either he or Mary had to remain at all times to magnetize and anchor the spiritual currents of the Christian Dispensation. Also left behind were Andrew, Mark, and Martha. Among the people making the journey were Peter, James, Bartholomew, Nathaniel, Mary of Bethany, and Pilate's wife, who was returning to Rome.

It was a small, but dedicated group of persons. Before leaving in the morning they all knelt in prayer. John gave the benediction, and the presence of Jesus was felt.

After the boat anchored in Alexandria, Mary, Peter, James and a few others went to Luxor. Here Mary extended her gratitude to the Hierarch, Serapis Bey, for the assistance received in bringing about Jesus' victory.

From Alexandria, the party decided to sail for Crete. Here the group magnetized the currents for the future visit by the Apostle Paul (now the Ascended Master Hilarion).

Then the boat headed for Rome, to have the wife of Pilate disembark. However, Jesus appeared and warned them not to go to Rome because of the existing hostile sentiment against Christians in that city. So the boat sailed on toward the Straits of Gibraltar.

At the southern tip of the Iberian Peninsula, Mary and others disembarked. Their journey would lead them through Portugal, Spain and France, and through the cities of Fatima, Lourdes and Orleans. Throughout the trip, Mary was in a constant state of listening grace. Sometimes she heard a delicate burst of music when crossing the aura of an individual whom she was to invite to accompany her party. In Portugal, she drew those who were later to be the children of Fatima, and from France she drew a small child who was later to become Bernadette. All of these joined the ever-growing group of travelers. The currents anchored at

Fatima, Lourdes and Orleans would be vitalized several hundred years later. During that later time when Mary appeared in Her luminous presence at Fatima and Lourdes, many healings, visitations, and contacts with children were made possible by the previous anchoring of spiritual currents. The children who saw Mary accepted Her Presence. Mary explained that the limited consciousness of the children made it impossible for Her to explain more of the Law.

Crossing the Pyrenees was difficult. It was done partially on foot and partially by donkey. When the group arrived in northern France, they re-united with Joseph of Arimathea, and together they crossed the channel.

After their arrival in Great Britain, Mary carried the Cup ashore. Overcome by a feeling of gratitude, they knelt in the sands. As they were kneeling, Jesus manifested Himself and gave the first benediction and ceremony of the "Holy Grail." Into this etheric record King Arthur of the Round Table later tuned in.

The Cup was left at Glastonbury. Here Mary and her group stayed for a while, making certain records for a future day.

Mary and her group remained in England for some time. They enjoyed their stay here. This country was destined to have a great future. Later Francis Bacon (now the Ascended Master Saint Germain) desired to establish a "United States of Europe," hoping, if it were successful, to extend it to the remainder of the world. Here, also, Jesus gave a blessing through radiation.

Mary and her group, with the exception of three individuals who stayed in England, traveled north to Wales and Scotland. Then they sailed to Ireland.

Here Mary met a young boy, who in a later embodiment, as Saint Patrick, helped establish Christianity in Ireland. The boy became a member of Mary's party.

Following their stay in Ireland, Mary's group

started their return home. The rough seas off the shores of Spain tossed the boat around. It was also not easy to travel with the small children who were aboard on the return trip. There was little room on the boat. Yet, considering there were many comparative strangers on board, Mary and her group had a harmonious journey home, sailing again through the Mediterranean.

At home after the long journey, Mary found that through Martha's care the household had run smoothly. Other things were pretty well disorganized. John, through his love, had held the group together in harmony, but he was also a dreamer, and had allowed many individual liberties. Things were in such disorder that Peter vowed never to go away again unless James could remain and be in charge rather than John.

MARY, THE PEACEMAKER

When reflecting upon the fifteen-year time span between the journey to Britain and her ascension, Mary called it the "fifteen most difficult years." These were difficult times because people of different backgrounds and personalities had to make the necessary adjustments caused by having to live together in close quarters. It was up to Mary to be the leader and referee. While assuming this position of spiritual leadership, it is clear from reading the original notes, that Mary never exhibited herself as a strong leader. Her function was to give general direction only, which may be compared to the task of an ombudsman, who gives opinions when asked.

One day Peter approached Mary, pointing out that most of the Christian community was still celebrating Jewish holidays, that it was high time to put into practice Jesus' teachings, and to establish some Christian holidays. Mary agreed, and Christmas was the first Christian holy day that was celebrated at Bethany. The disciples prepared a small crib as a surprise for Mary, and the birth of Jesus was re-enacted. The celebration of Easter, Jesus' Ascension Day, and Pentecost, followed.

Another time Peter burst into Mary's room very upset. He stated that some "heathens from India" had just painted a sun over the newly white-washed walls of the house, and were worshipping it. Mary investigated and found a large sun, symbolic of Osiris. She explained that the sun was to these people a symbol of life, and they were honoring a symbol without worshipping it, in the same way that the disciples were honoring Jesus without worshipping him. Mary then asked Peter to get together with Andrew and white-wash over the Osiris-symbol. Mary offered to give the men from India some sunflower seeds. They could be planted against the house, and the sunflowers could serve as a symbol of the sun. Everyone was pleased with this compromise.

Some other folks from India also caused problems. They sat all day in the corner of the courtyard and did not move from that position. The disciples had an understanding that everyone who was going to share the food had to make a contribution to the overall work load of the community. There was some resentment against the men from the far East sitting all day doing nothing. Again Mary came to the rescue. She explained to the disciples that these men had come very far just to get the radiation of Jesus, which was the "hem of his garment." They, on the other hand, had had the privilege of living with and knowing Jesus while he was on this plane. The disciples were satisfied, and gave the men from India all types of food, more than they wished for.

Often, after the disciples and the apostles had

returned from their long journeys, they found that the hot sands had cracked their feet. So, Mary, with the help of Mary Magdalene, created an ointment that quickly healed them. Mary Magdalene was much interested in perfume. Peter did not like it and asked Mary to do something about this worldly practice. Again Mary acted as a peacemaker. She suggested putting the perfume into the foot ointment. Everyone thought this was a good idea.

There were the tests and trials of daily living. There were also happy times, when visitors from many parts of the world arrived; there were the happy communions of Mary and John at the top of the hill at Bethany, and there were what Mary called "the other sort of experiences."

Whenever Jesus approached, the melody of "Joy to the World" was heard by Mary and some of the disciples. This had already occurred at a time right after the resurrection. Mary said the melody was so distinctive, she wondered why all of the disciples couldn't hear it.

Some nights Peter, Andrew and James had words. Andrew and James wanted a change of routine. They longed for the fresh breezes of the Sea of Galilee, and they wanted to go there to fish. Peter was opposed to this. Mary suggested to go together, preach the Gospel, and to give up fishing, for now they were all "fishers of men." All three agreed and walked arm in arm to Galilee.

One day the lovely wife of Pilate came to Mary, complaining that Peter had chopped the head off a statue that represented Apollo. When Peter was asked why he did it, he said that he didn't think Roman gods had any place in the community. Mary asked Peter to restore the head, since the figure only represented love and beauty.

Mary, through her training prior to this embodiment, had some experience with elementals. She knew that bees respond to certain sounds. Mary attracted the bees with the sound of clinking brassware. This way everybody had honey to go with the unleavened bread.

John gradually assumed the likeness of Jesus. The shine of his hair, the brilliance of his face, even the contour of his face became like his Master. According to the Masters, when Jesus communicated with Mary and John on top of the hill of Bethany, the method of conveyance was almost identical to that of the Masters who spoke through the messenger, Geraldine Innocenti, in the 1950's. John wrote down his revelations, which do not coincide with the revelations printed in today's Bible. In the 1950's John applied to the Karmic Board for a dispensation that would permit him to give his revelations again, using the words as he recorded them at the time when he was a disciple of Jesus.

When Saul of Tarsus (Paul) came to Bethany, he suffered great remorse over what he had done to a Christian, named Stephens, and others. He also regretted very much not having been in a state of "listening grace," thereby missing his opportunity to be part of Jesus' ministry. Paul consecrated the remainder of his life to making amends. This he did, but there were temporary setbacks. Sometimes one could find him in the depths of despair, with tears running down his cheeks. At other times he would display the arrogance of his earlier life. He would argue violently with the disciples who did not have formal training. When things started to get out of hand, Mary stepped in. She reminded Paul that he should listen to the disciples because they had been a witness to Jesus' ministry, and had lived in his aura. Then, Paul relented.

True to his previous statement, Peter never went on a mission unless he was sure James would remain at Bethany.

MARY'S ASCENSION

About nine years before the close of her embodiment, Mary asked Peter to build a small house and chapel apart from the community to help her to work out her ascension. This was done, and Mary spent the remainder of her life at this accommodation, located at the edge of the stream that ran through the area. Mary of Bethany and other friends supplied her with flowers, candles, and fresh fruit.

After some time, it became physically difficult for Mary to make the daily climb of the hill at Bethany with John for the meeting with Jesus. Therefore, John now undertook this task alone. One year, in the month of May, Mary asked John to call the disciples together. She knew that before the end of August she would join Jesus.

It took considerable time for all of the disciples to return home. Some stayed at places as far away as Greece. Before all of them arrived, Mary asked the community to build a very simple chapel on top of the hill of Bethany for her.

On August 10, Mary walked up the hill alone, following the very path Jesus had trod many years before. She remained in the newly-built chapel for three days, praying and fasting. Then the disciples joined her, all of them having arrived home by this time.

Together they walked down the hill to Mary's home. Here she spoke to them and to the original disciples particularly. She told them that on August 15 her ascension would be completed, and she asked them how they wished to pursue the remainder of their lives while in this embodiment.

John said that he would follow her as soon as he

heard the voice of his Presence telling him that it was time. Paul said that he would do the same thing. He added that if the ascension were offered to him, he would take the opportunity at once. Knowing his own nature, he would take no chances asking for a postponement. (Under Cosmic law, it is possible to delay the ascension. The date of the ascension then depends upon the individual's own wishes, and upon his performance in life. If there should be additional karma, it is possible that the ascension would have to be delayed until some future embodiment.)

Peter, James, and Andrew took a different position. They said, "We shall endeavor to continue throughout the Christian Dispensation, Mother, what you have done throughout these thirty years."

Mary blessed the disciples. Next, the other members of the community entered. She blessed them also. Then she closed her eyes to this world. Her body was placed inside a rocky tomb, and the tomb was sealed for three days.

When Mary awoke beyond the veil, she met Joseph first, and then Jesus. Afterwards she prepared for the ascension of her physical form. Mary raised the vibrations of her flesh form, and absorbed the purified physical body into her Christ-Self. Then she entered consciously into the heart of her I AM Presence, as Jesus had done before her. In the tomb she placed one white rose for each member of the community.

When the door was rolled back from Mary's tomb, they found the body was gone, and there was the fragrance of the roses.

Thereafter Mary enjoyed the renewing of her association with all those precious individuals who had assisted her call from the other side, namely Lord Maitreya, Archangels Gabriel and Raphael, Jesus and Joseph, and John the Baptist.

Words will never be sufficient to express our gratitude to those most precious Beings, Jesus and Mary. Perhaps their life accomplishments during their last embodiment on earth may best be summed up by quoting the words of the beloved Lord Krishna: "Service is the Law of Life!"

10 - The Time Period From Jesus To 1961

THE KNIGHTS OF THE ROUND TABLE

The Great White Brotherhood held their first council at Shamballa many thousands of years ago. They joined together around a glorious round golden table. Sanat Kumara was the presiding Master. To each member he gave certain responsibilities, according to the nature of the individúal. At certain intervals the council met, and each reported on the expansion of the service in his particular field. All rejoiced in every development that brought the purpose of the Brotherhood to greater manifestation, but none interfered with the specific services of the other.

As certain members of the human race were attracted toward the spiritual center of Shamballa, they were invited to attend these councils in their inner bodies, and to participate in the discussions. King Arthur's Order of the Round Table was conceived when an illuminated lifestream tuned into the etheric record of Shamballa and created a focus for God in the outer world. This happened in the fourth century (A.D.). The now Ascended Master Saint Germain was then embodied as Merlin, the Magician, and the now Ascended Master El Morya was embodied as King Arthur. The Knights of the Round Table were the oarsmen, who in a former embodiment had carried the "Sacred Cup" to Britain with Mary.

The quest for the Holy Grail by King Arthur's knights was the search for the consciousness of the Christ. The Grail signifies inspired consciousness into which is poured the Divine Will. The diamond spear signifies the projecting forth of the energy into action and accomplishment. Looking at today's conditions, many in the East have completed the action of the Grail, but it is to the Western consciousness that the Masters look for the manifestation of the spear, through the release of constructive, vital energies of individuals.

As was pointed out previously when discussing the Christian Dispensation, every 100 years within the 2000-year cycle the Lords of Karma give a dispensation of energy to the spiritual Hierarchy of the Earth. The Being known as the Lord of the World (now Gautama Buddha), the World Teacher, and the Maha Chohan, in council decide how best to invest that energy. They look upon the requirements of Cosmic Law. They look upon Earth conditions, and they look upon individuals of sufficient spiritual growth to assume a role among the persons embodied. Then they present a plan to the entire Great White Brotherhood. Opportunity is offered to some Masters and their embodied chelas. The final outcome of the plan depends entirely upon the voluntary choice of the chela, since the Masters have to respect the free will of the students.

From the year 1300 until the beginning of the 17th century, this impersonal energy was given primarily to the Master Saint Germain to bring forth a new land (America) to the minds of the people in Europe, and to create the cradle for the future spiritual endeavor which is to flourish under the Seventh Ray. "Prompted by vital energies and a quality called the love of freedom, Columbus and other explorers left home and security to face an unknown course, a chartless sea and carved out a continent upon which rests the future of the civilized world."

"Men of destiny are swept by the Cosmic Mind of the Holy Spirit. They are carried by a pressure that governs their outer consciousness." They are the wayshowers; they are the hope of the Earth. For countless centuries the Great White Brotherhood has sponsored such efforts and served the human race, without more than a handful of people being cognizant of their very existence. In spite of being assisted by Divine Beings, the lives of these embodied way-showers hardly ever was an easy one. "Men and women of destiny always had to suffer the resistance and ridicule of the human race." They had to bear the cross; "they had to strain at the gnat and swallow the camel to fulfill their mission. Today it is no different."

AN OVERVIEW OF THE LIVES OF VARIOUS ASCENDED BEINGS

Serapis Bey

Serapis Bey is a guardian spirit who is assisting the Earth. He was a priest in the Ascension Temple of Atlantis. Just before the sinking of Poseidonis, he entered a boat and, together with 39 other volunteers, transferred the Ascension Flame to Luxor. Here Serapis Bey established a Temple for the Ascension Flame, and has been its principal guardian ever since. Some trusted brother took Serapis′ place when he was at inner levels during embodiments, or when he was in embodiment in another country. Most of Serapis Bey′s embodiments took place in Egypt.

As Phidias, an Athenian architect and sculptor, he designed the Parthenon and supervised its construction.

According to A.D.K. Luk, his embodiments also included that of Akhenaton IV, King Leonidas of Sparta, and Amenophis III. In the latter embodiment he built the temples at Thebes and Karnak. The date of his ascension is given as around 400 B.C.

Serapis Bey is now the Chohan of the Fourth Ray. He leads the Brotherhood at Luxor and works with the Seraphim.

Every lifestream emits a series of tones called a

keynote. This keynote is normally contained in a known musical composition. The keynotes of about 40 Masters and retreats were given by the Masters to the students. The keynote of a retreat is usually that of its Hierarch. Next to having a picture of a Master — these were also given — a keynote is an effective way to tune in and make a connection to inner realms with a Master. The keynote for Serapis Bey is contained in the melody "Celeste Aida."

El Morya

The Ascended Master El Morya came to Earth as a guardian spirit from Mercury.

El Morya was a king in many embodiments. During the birth of Jesus he was Melchior, one of the "three wise men." The other wise men were the now Ascended Masters Kuthumi and Djwal Kul.

El Morya was King Arthur of the fifth and sixth centuries. In order to soften his nature and give a better balance after his many embodiments as a king, he embodied as Sir Thomas Moore, the poet.

A.D.K. Luk states that El Morya led three crusades, and was a Rajput king of India. Continuing this account, El Morya retained the body of his last incarnation for 325 years before making His ascension around 1888. This statement appears to be correct, because the dictations of the Masters explain that El Morya "used the etheric body of an Indian potentate during his association with H. Blavatsky."

El Morya is Chief of the Council of the Great White Brotherhood in India, and is in charge of the retreat located near Darjeeling. His disciplines are very strict. He is known for his ability to get things done without taking detours. Chelaship under this

Master may be compared to clawing one's way up a sheer cliff, sustaining cuts and bruises, but arriving there comparatively quickly.

Together with the Ascended Master Saint Germain, El Morya was able to obtain a dispensation under which additional information concerning Cosmic Law, retreats and historical data could be given through the messenger Geraldine Innocenti, his twin-flame. This happened from 1952 through August 1961.

El Morya is the Chohan of the First Ray, and gives assistance to all that are desirous of doing God's will. His keynote is "Panis Angelicus."

Hilarion

Hilarion was a priest in the Temple of Truth on Atlantis. Before Poseidonis sank, he volunteered to bring the Flame of Truth to Crete. Crete at that time was a part of Greece. Hilarion arrived at Crete just before Poseidonis sank.

With the assistance of Pallas Athena, the Goddess of Truth, Hilarion and the other priests built the Temple of Truth on Crete. This took many embodiments.

The focus of truth later brought forth the oracles of Delphi, who functioned for hundreds of years. The people had faith in the Delphic Order, but eventually fell prey to the actions of a few oracles and priests who allowed themselves to be bought. Finally, the Masters had to withdraw.

In Biblical times, Hilarion was known as Saul of Tarsus, and later as the Apostle Paul. Saul had a certain set belief as to how the Messiah would come. This caused him to miss seeing Jesus. Saul was on the way to Damascus when Jesus — after His ascension — appeared to him. That visitation changed Saul's life.

Much of his arrogance and pride was consumed. He became known as the Apostle Paul. He suffered much remorse for having missed Jesus, while Jesus was in physical embodiment.

Later on, Hilarion had an embodiment as the philosopher Iamblichus.

According to A.D.K. Luk, Hilarion's last embodiment was spent in a town near Gaza [now known as a city on the "Gaza Strip," captured by Israel]. This occurred about 300 A.D. He was educated at Alexandria. Afterwards he lived as a hermit in the desert, directing a great number of students. He ascended from the earthly plane at a place among almost inaccessible rocks. Hilarion is now Chohan of the Fifth Ray, the ray of science, healing and truth. He will assist anyone who sincerely wants to know truth. Healing is another of his interests. He enjoys assisting medical researchers in alleviating pain and suffering. Finally, He likes to assist skeptics, atheists and the disillusioned. He is very successful in again instilling in them a faith in God.

His keynote is "Onward Christian Soldiers."

Nada

Nada was the Ascended Master who assisted Saint Germain in obtaining the dispensation that made it possible to bring about the instructions by various Ascended Beings after 1930, through the messenger, Guy W. Ballard. The dictations state, "Saint Germain and Nada stood alone."

On Atlantis, Nada served in the "Temple of Divine Love," located where New Bedford, Massachusetts now is. From that temple, healing rays were directed all over the globe to those who needed and desired them.

Nada, in her last embodiment on Earth, entered the retreat at Luxor. Here she received the rigorous disciplines of the Ascension Temple. In the beginning she found it very difficult to maintain harmony during her training, with the frictions and the various human qualities that need to be overcome when living in close association with other students. She told the students in the 1930's that sometimes she left the retreat and ran miles through the desert, just to get away from the pressures.

Nada made the ascension in about 700 B.C. Healing is one of her actions of service to mankind. She is also ready to give assistance to individuals who desire help in overcoming bad habits such as drinking and smoking.

One can feel more comfortable when experiencing cold temperatures by asking to be enfolded in Her pink flame of love.

Nada is a member of the Karmic Board, representing the Third Ray, the ray of love. She is also the Chohan of the Sixth Ray. Her keynote is found in the song "I Love You Truly" from the "Chocolate Soldier."

Kuthumi

Kuthumi's first-mentioned embodiment was that of Pythagoras (500 B.C.). He established a school at Crotona, in southern Italy, where he made important discoveries in several fields — mathematics, astronomy, and music.

According to A.D.K. Luk, he determined that the world was round, that the planets produced the "Music of the Spheres," and that man's real self is immortal, and that he has to come back into embodiment repeatedly, until making the ascension.

In Biblical times he was Balthazar, one of the three wise men. He could have ascended then, but postponed his ascension, as El Morya did, in order to bring forth Theosophy.

Later on, Kuthumi embodied as Saint Francis of Assissi (about 1200 A.D.). He was a great lover of animals, and helped thousands of them to the point where they did not have to come back into embodiment. Kuthumi was a very patient and gentle man. He could spend hours or an entire day observing a flower come into full bloom.

In a later embodiment Kuthumi built the Taj Mahal in India (1640 A.D.), one of the world's most beautiful buildings.

In his last embodiment, he and El Morya were instrumental in bringing forth Theosophy. "Kuthumi maintained one embodiment in India for 300 years, and ascended from a valley in the Himalayan Mountains in about 1889" (A.D.K. Luk).

His keynote is found in the "Kashmiri Song." (Pale Hands I Loved.)

Saint Germain

With the possible exception of Jesus and Mary, more information is known about Saint Germain than any other Ascended Being. The following is a brief summary of his various embodiments. Students desiring additional information on this subject may read *Law of Life* by A.D.K. Luk, or *The Comte de Saint Germain* by I. Cooper-Oakley.

Saint Germain's endeavors to free mankind started during the "Sahara Civilization," 70,000 years ago. He could have gained his ascension at that time, but he chose to re-embody many times in order to maintain a better connection to the Earth by keeping a physical body. He retained continuity of consciousness during the remainder of his embodiments.

In another embodiment Saint Germain was a priest in the "Temple of Purification" near today's Cuba.

In about the eleventh century B.C., Saint Germain embodied as the Prophet Samuel. According to A.D.K. Luk, the term "Uncle Sam" refers to that embodiment of Saint Germain.

As Joseph, together with Mary, Saint Germain prepared the way for Jesus. He knew of Jesus' mission in advance, and in this way was able to help with his training. Jesus, as a young man visited India. Here he made contact with the Ascended Being known as The Great Divine Director, and received the keywords for his mission, "I am the Resurrection and the Life." Thereafter, Joseph's mission was accomplished. At the time of his passing, he determined to give assistance to all human beings and animals, in making their passing an easy one, provided he would receive such a call.

As the Greek philosopher Proclus (450 A.D.), Saint Germain had a school in Athens. He traveled much, and taught various religions. Later on he became Merlin, the magician of King Arthur's Court.

A.D.K. Luk states that Saint Germain embodied as Roger Bacon (approximately 1211 to 1294 A.D.). Bacon was an English monk and philosopher, who made several scientific discoveries. He also produced an elixir to prolong life. Next, in the fourteenth century, followed an embodiment in Germany as Christian Rosenkreutz. Translated, Rosenkreutz means "Cross of Roses." After undergoing several initiations in Egypt, Rosenkreutz returned to Germany. There he founded the "Order of the Rosy Cross," of which today's Rosicrucian Order is an offspring.

Continuing with the account of A.D.K. Luk, Saint Germain's next embodiments were as Christopher

Columbus and Paracelsus, a Swiss chemist and physician.

Saint Germain's last embodiment was that of Francis Bacon, an English philosopher and writer. He wrote several books, including the plays by William Shakespeare. The name Will-i-am signifies that according to the will of the "I AM" (God), Francis Bacon would shake the spear of wisdom at a world full of darkness and ignorance. (This was Saint Germain's special activity, namely the illumination of every age in which he chose an embodiment.) There are some 500 instances in which the name Francis Bacon is written in acrostic cypher code in the Shakespearean plays. He also wrote a book on cypher code, which is still used as a reference in this field.

It is generally believed that Francis Bacon passed on in 1626. However, this is not so. Attending his own funeral dressed as a woman, he let it appear that way. Thereafter, Francis Bacon left England and traveled to Transylvania. He left the earth plane on May 1, 1684, ascending on the Freedom Flame, a flame He had nurtured for centuries.

After His ascension, Saint Germain appeared again in Europe. According to A.D.K. Luk and I. Cooper-Oakley, He was known as the Comte de Saint Germain in France, as the Wonderman and Prince Rakoczy in Germany, and as Comte Bellamarre in Venice. Wherever Saint Germain went, He was considered very wealthy. He made it appear that way in order to gain influence among the heads of government. The overall plan was to use that influence as a means of effecting change — change in bringing about greater harmony and cooperation between the nations of Europe.

Saint Germain returned in his visible, tangible, Ascended Master Body, just prior to the French Revolution and would have prevented it had the people listened to His counsel. Through his association with the Court of France, he attempted to externalize a

United States of Europe as early as the 18th Century, during the reign of Louis XVI and Marie Antoinette.

It was Saint Germain who inspired the people of Oberammergau to give the Passion Play every ten years, in gratitude to God for relief from the plague.

Saint Germain protected and encouraged those responsible for America's freedom. The inception of this country was due largely to His tireless efforts. The drafting of the Declaration of Independence was also a direct result of His assistance. As an unknown visitor, Saint Germain made a fiery speech, urging the people assembled, to "Sign that document!" Afterwards He could not be found, although the doors had been locked and guarded.

Saint Germain provided the guidance which sustained Washington and Lincoln during their darkest hours.

During the time El Morya and Kuthumi brought forth Theosophy, Saint Germain was not active. He was preparing for a future time period when He would work together with Nada on a special dispensation given shortly before 1930. After being granted that dispensation, Saint Germain worked with the first messenger, Mr. Guy W. Ballard, until Mr. Ballard transitioned in 1939. This time Saint Germain used a new approach. Instead of attempting to try to impress people with His wealth, he used a method of instruction based upon logic and common sense. In addition He added His radiation, which helped the instruction gain acceptance through the feeling nature of the students. Other Ascended Masters and students joined this effort, which was called the "I AM Activity."

After Mr. Ballard's transition, Saint Germain, together with El Morya, was able to obtain another dispensation. This happened in about 1950, and through this effort, called "The Bridge to Freedom," additional information concerning Cosmic Law, Masters, retreats, and the divine plan for the Earth could be given. The name of the second messenger was Geraldine

Innocente. This effort continued until August of 1961, when Geraldine transitioned.

Saint Germain's retreat is the Rakoczy Mansion in Transylvania. He has a focus in the Etheric City over the Sahara Desert.

The electronic pattern of Saint Germain's lifestream is the Maltese cross. His keynote and the keynote of His retreat in Transylvania are contained in the Strauss waltzes. The Ascended Master Teaching Foundation uses "Emperor's Waltz" as His keynote and the keynote of His retreat. A.D.K. Luk uses the same melody as the keynote of His retreat.

For about 180 years, Saint Germain has been the Chohan of the Seventh Ray. On May 1, 1954 He assumed responsibility as a director for the new cycle of the 2000-year period of the Seventh Ray. This gave Him additional authority to increase the understanding of the qualities of this ray. Jesus was the director of the past 2000-year-cycle, when the Sixth Ray was predominant.

THE THEOSOPHICAL SOCIETY

The Masters provided us with an in-depth look as to how the Theosophical Society was perceived at inner realms, how the plan was put into operation, who were its principal participants were, and what caused the downfall of the Masters' first attempt to acquaint mankind on a larger scale than here-to-fore with a knowledge of Cosmic Law and the activities of the Great White Brotherhood.

Early in the 19th Century Lord Maitreya (Jesus' teacher) called the attention of the Chohans (Lords of the Rays) of the Earth to the necessity of bringing the knowledge of the actual existence of the Masters to the outer consciousness of the people. He explained that here-to-fore the Masters had concentrated their attention upon the East, and it was time to shift such attention to the occidental world.

"The universal presence of the Holy Ones had long been accepted in the East. However, the absolute disregard for form — they wanted essence, not form — and the nature of the Eastern Holy Man, being absolutely devoted and limited to adoration and worship, did not allow for the use of the vital energies required to translate vision into tangible action and results.

"Lord Maitreya in his pleasant, persuasive and eloquent manner, continued in His presentation, and outlined what is known today as Theosophy. He explained to the Chohans how certain lifestreams might embody and then those Masters who felt close to them could step through the veil and convince the people of the reality of the Masters.

"The conditions of the Causal Bodies of thousands indicated that many individuals were qualified to render a service. Blavatsky, Leadbeater, Olcott, Besant and Judge were among these. After a good deal of effort and persuasion by the Masters, Mrs. Blavatsky offered her assistance." Mrs. Blavatsky, in turn, attempted to gain the support of Mr. Olcott. It was not, however, until the Master El Morya took off his turban and showed it to Mr. Olcott as proof, that he was a real, tangible being, that Mr. Olcott agreed. El Morya added, saying to the students, "For me, I would say that was quite a concession." The Theosophical Society was founded in 1875.

El Morya explained that Messrs. Leadbeater, Judge, Sinnett and many others were perhaps better qualified than Helen Blavatsky, but they did not volunteer for leadership. Mrs. Blavatsky stood forth and said, "Masters, I will go and be that wedge." El Morya continued, stating that, generally speaking, out of thousands of qualified lifestreams, perhaps ten are willing to volunteer. Out of those ten, one will be chosen, and the Masters' hopes rest on that particular lifestream.

In spite of being somewhat undeveloped and "rough in body, mind, spirit, and soul" Helen Blavatsky qualified because she had several previous embodiments of cooperative service with the Masters. She also had the faculty of advanced clairvoyance and clairaudience. These faculties the Masters El Morya and Kuthumi accelerated, to communicate with her. During the entire association with Helen Blavatsky the Masters used the etheric body of an Indian potentate. Certain instructions also were given to Mrs. Blavatsky at the Luxor Retreat. Upon receiving this instruction, and after passing the initiation of the first and second temples, Helen proceeded to the third temple. It is the task of the third temple to bring the student together with six other students who have within them the particular nature and characteristics which irk the student. People resist persons, places, conditions, and things because they have not mastered themselves. Adjusting to these six individuals is not an easy task, and requires exceptional tolerance and love. Most students do not pass this test. Helen Blavatsky did not pass it either; she left the third temple and did not return. These tests are no longer given in retreats. Since 1930, when the occult law was set aside, they are presented in the outer world, in every-day life activities.

The outpouring through the Theosophical Society occurred primarily through the Second Ray of Wisdom. El Morya, Kuthumi, Serapis Bey and the Maha Chohan poured through the mind of Helen Blavatsky the wisdom which she wrote into the *Secret Doctrine*, the *Voice of Isis*, and the other volumes, many of which are yet secreted in the Masters′ retreats. It was the same truth that was contained in the *Vedas* and *Upanishads*.

The Maha Chohan, Kuthumi, and El Morya released to Helen Blavatsky the powers of precipitation and phenomena, to captivate, convince and please the senses of the students. However, the curiosity seekers were never satisfied, no matter how much phenomena was produced, and they sooner or later returned to an easier field of study.

Hundreds of letters were written, many by the Masters "K.H." (Kuthumi) and "M." (El Morya) to A.P. Sinnett and A.O. Hume. These were later compiled into the book *The Mahatma Letters to A.P. Sinnett*.

Some students of Theosophy distorted the works of the Masters by resorting to spiritualism. The dark forces seized upon spiritualism and concocted all kinds of materializing seances, trumpet seances, and other schemes to bring the people into darkness.

The members of the Theosophical Society were mostly content to confine their energies to an interest in the new knowledge, and except in rare instances, contributed little of their own energies in expiating the karma of the race by giving impersonal service. In other words, the students did not return a balance for the new knowledge received, and after some time the energy allowed to the Masters was depleted. The Masters said they learned from this experience, and it made them more cautious in the investment of their energy, proceeding thenceforth to procure the greatest good and the fullest manifestation of an endeavor before the energy ran out. This is why, during the next dispensation, they showed the students how to return the energies to effect even greater accomplishment.

OTHER MESSENGERS OF THE BROTHERHOOD

In addition to Helen Blavatsky, there were other individuals, who in the 19th and 20th centuries, gave certain new phases of the teachings of the Great White Brotherhood to mankind. The Masters mentioned Joseph Smith, Mary Baker Eddy, Alice Bailey, Baird Spaulding, Guy W. Ballard and Geraldine Innocenti. [Mrs. Eddy was the author of *Science and Health with Key to the Scriptures*, and other books. She stressed spiritual healing, in the way Jesus healed the sick, and called her discovery of the healing method "Christian Science."]

Alice Bailey and Baird Spaulding [through his books *Life and Teaching of the Masters of the Far East*] carried to the western mind a greater realization of the activities of the Ascended Masters. In 1919 Djwal Kul obtained a dispensation enabling him to speak to Alice Bailey. She was a "natural" automatic writer, but did not seek, at first, the opportunity to be a medium. It took great persuasion before she finally consented. Djwal Kul and Alice Bailey had a close association during some previous time period. This was helpful in obtaining the dispensation.

Another messenger needs to be mentioned here. This individual called himself "the Hermit." His spiritual name was "Brother Amo," his real name remains a mystery. Wounded in the Franco-Prussian War, Brother Amo decided to go India to obtain a healing. Having arrived here he found himself expected, and he was guided to a retreat in the high Himalayas. After many years and after undergoing many tests and initiations, Brother Amo completed the final initiation into the Great White Brotherhood. All this happened at the beginning of the twentieth century. Later on, he left the Himalayas and settled near a small village in the state of Wyoming. He wrote about his experiences in the book *Die Mitteilungen des Eremiten*, (The Explanations of a Hermit). Before leaving this plane of existence, Brother Amo promised the author of the book, Felix Schmidt, that he would communicate with him from beyond the veil.

After several years had gone by, Felix Schmidt started to find, among his manuscripts (he was a writer), written messages from Brother Amo. This continued until 1951. The messages from "the other side" were compiled by Felix Schmidt in the book *Kundgebungen des Eremiten*, (Messages from a Hermit.) While both books stress the important spiritual task Germans should fulfill as part of the Divine Plan for the Earth, the descriptions of every-day-life in a retreat, the explanations of some aspects of the Law (for example how to recognize a "true prophet"), and his detailed descriptions of the world beyond the physical scene of life are unique, and should be of interest to many.

THE FIRST "NEW AGE" DISPENSATION

The Dawn of a New Era

The first "New Age" dispensation was primarily the effort of the Ascended Master Saint Germain. He sought out those who had assisted Him in his previous efforts with the Sahara Civilization 70,000 years ago, and saw enough reason to carry the light to America and the people of the Earth. The Ascended Lady Master Nada assisted the efforts of Saint Germain.

This new dispensation shows an entirely new approach. It reminds one of the statement by Brother Amo that any new religious teaching is designed to meet the needs of the hour and the progress of the human race, is given at a particular part of the globe and presented to a pre-designated group of people. Saint Germain did not use as a foundation any established religious teaching, using it as a base and adding to it. He and other Ascended Masters made no attempt to receive Theosophy, only sparingly did They refer to the *Bible*, only in rare instances did They refer to the Vedic literature of India. Starting totally anew, without relying on previous teachings, Saint Germain and other Ascended Masters explained Cosmic Law in clear terms. The method of instruction was based on logic and common sense. In addition, the Masters added Their radiation, which helped the instruction gain acceptance through the feeling nature of the students. Saint Germain gave out this new message in America, which at this particular time period is to be the leader of the human race and He presented to the world a new style of Ascended Master Teaching.

There were changes in the substance of the teaching as well. As part of the dispensation, the occult law was set aside, mainly as a result of the peril the Earth is in. For the first time since the sinking of Atlantis, the Ascended Master could give the knowledge of the I AM Presence and the Violet Flame in public. (The Violet Flame erases the karma of the past.) Before this time it was only permitted to be given in retreats, to people of considerable spiritual advancement.

For these reasons, commencing with this dispensation, Ascended Master Teaching did assume a new approach, unique from any other previous method of instruction and this effort by Saint Germain has been labeled by the Masters the "beginning of a new age."

When Saint Germain first conceived the idea of putting forth this work, he explained to the Master called the Great Divine Director, that he had two people in embodiment (Mr. and Mrs. G.W. Ballard), who he felt were strong enough to carry His message. The Great Divine Director asked him if he were certain of this. Saint Germain replied, "I shall try it out, and we shall see!"

The messenger, Guy W. Ballard, met Saint Germain first in August of 1930 on Mount Shasta. This historical, illuminating experience is beautifully detailed in the book *Unveiled Mysteries*, by Godfré Ray King. After the experiences on Mt. Shasta, Mr. Ballard returned to his house in Chicago, where further explanations were given him by Saint Germain as part of many discourses. These instructions were given to the Ballards via the light ray and the sound ray. Some were delivered by Saint Germain in his Ascended Master Body.

The "eyewitness" told me the experiences of an employee of the Ballards. The governess told the eyewitness that she knew Saint Germain would be contacting the Ballards, and, not wanting to be in the way, left the home. While walking down the street it suddenly began to rain on her side of the street only. That made her go back because she then realized she should be present as a witness to that which was going on. This she did.

Following this period of preparation, the work of the "I AM Activity" was started in 1934. Mr. Ballard gave classes, and talked to large audiences all over the United States. Mrs. Ballard talked over the radio. Together they reached hundreds of thousands of people.

Saint Germain was lavish in his praise of Mr. and Mrs. Ballard. He said: "They have proven their ability to stand in the Light, and with no personal desire, unselfishly carry the pure unadulterated message of the MIGHTY I AM PRESENCE. It is only through their joyous and willing obedience to our slightest wish, that it is possible to bring forth this expression and understanding of the I AM in purity and clearness." Mr. and Mrs. Ballard had earned this high calling of being authorized messengers of the Great White Brotherhood by being associated with Saint Germain in various embodiments. Mr. Ballard, in a previous embodiment, was George Washington, Mrs. Ballard had an embodiment as Benjamin Franklin, and another as Joan of Arc.

The "eyewitness" mentioned in the foreword followed the car caravan of the Ballards. She became a member of the staff, writing at one time a series of basic instructions for beginners. According to the "eyewitness," Mr. Ballard never knew what he was going to talk about. All he knew was that Saint Germain requested that he rent a certain auditorium in a certain city, on a certain date. After this was done and the audience was assembled, Mr. Ballard stepped to the platform. There appeared before him two-inch high letters of "golden living light." Those messages he read to the audience. Some people in the front row also saw those letters of light. According to A.D.K. Luk, Mr. Ballard was clairvoyant and clairaudient. Usually he had no problem reading the two inch letters to the public, but when he was disturbed, it was like reading through tears.

The Occult Law Explained

Cosmic Law does not change in fundamental principle, but in its application and result to mankind. It was about 80,000 years ago, during the time of Atlantis, that the occult law was introduced. Occult means hidden or veiled, and from that time until 1930 an explanation of the Law could only be given in a veiled manner, certain truths appearing as legends, myths, allegories and symbolism. In addition, information could be given only on a limited, gradual basis. In some cases, incorrect information was given out purposely. It was up to the student to ponder and evaluate the knowledge given.

Examples of literature coming under the occult law are Homer's *Illiad* (it contained the story of Troy), the *Bible*, the *Vedas*, Plato's dialogues given in *Critias* and *Timaeus*, and all published writings under Theosophy. To illustrate how things were veiled under the occult law, here are some quotations from *The Mahatma Letters to A.P. Sinnett*:

1) page 78 K.H.: "I have just been permitted, for the first time, to give you the right figure."
2) page 78 "The Monad performs not only 'world rings' or 7 major inmetalliations, inherbations, zoonisations? and incarnations — but an infinitude of subrings or subordinate whirls all in series of sevens."
3) page 79 "I am more than willing to help out, but things have to be divulged gradually." (gradually was written in italics). "I am sorry to refuse you, I cannot, am not permitted to answer your question."

There is another interesting point to consider. When an Ascended Master received a dispensation under the occult law, this became the deciding factor as far as the type of instruction was concerned. For instance, the Master Djwal Kul received the dispensation to work through Alice Bailey. This happened in 1919, a year when the occult law was still in effect. Mrs. Bailey received instructions until around 1949, when the occult law no longer applied. However, since the dispensation was received in 1919, Mrs. Bailey could not talk about certain items, such as the knowledge of the I AM Presence and the Violet Flame, even though this was already given to mankind in 1930, through Mr. Ballard.

The writings of Brother Amo fall into the same category. He received his training in a Retreat in the Himalayas in about 1900. Brother Amo first published his experiences in 1949. His writings contain unique details of life in a retreat and more than 90% of His book is written in a straightforward manner, without being veiled; however, his writings do not include the knowledge of the I AM Presence and the Violet Flame.

What enabled Mr. Ballard and Geraldine Innocenti to receive messages from the Masters in clear and simple terms, giving mankind, for the first time since the days of Atlantis, the knowledge of the I AM Presence and the Violet Flame? It was the need of the hour. Under the dispensation given to Saint Germain and Nada, instructions did not need to be veiled. Mysticism is no longer the requirement of the hour.

There was a good reason for the occult law. By talking in riddles and allegories many truth seekers escaped the wrath of fanatical priests, notably the ones of the so-called Christian Church. It was difficult to persecute people as heretics, if a great deal of what they said was subject to interpretation.

Accomplishments of the First Dispensation

With the introduction of the I AM Activity, the Masters for the first time placed emphasis upon the art of invocation. They explained that the students could best support their efforts if they would employ the power of the spoken word, called decreeing. The student body responded to this request, and this helped greatly to bring about a manifestation of the plan of the Great Ones.

Since the Masters indicated that decreeing is the key element in helping to usher in the Permanent Golden Age on Earth, this item will be discussed in further detail in Part III of this book.

Saint Germain said that without the calls (decrees) of the students, portions of the eastern and western coasts of the U.S. would have disappeared. Because of the student's efforts, additional protection could be given by the Masters. This happened in early 1936.

As part of this effort, the cities of New York and San Francisco were saved from destruction. The energy released by the students enabled Saint Germain to create a vertical line of protection along the eastern and western seaboards of North America. It also made it possible for Saint Germain to release tremendous power through the messengers, which helped to bring the destructive efforts under control.

"The call of the students in cooperation with Elohim Cyclopea, the All-Seeing-Eye, directing currents of energy, prevented a tidal wave from striking the west coast of the United States. This was to have come into effect on January 2, 1936." (Saint Germain, February, 1936)

"The devastation that was planned for America would have begun more than 18 months ago had it not been for the tremendous release of power by Saint Germain through the messengers." (Goddess of Liberty, December 5, 1937)

What was the outer cause of this destruction the Masters talked about? There were several warnings about the destruction of BOTH coasts. An earthquake in the Pacific Ocean could be responsible for a tidal wave striking the west coast only. The same holds true for a quake occurring in the Atlantic Ocean. It would not effect the West Coast. The chances of a quake occurring simultaneously in the Pacific and the Atlantic are slim, since there are no known gas belts crossing the United States.

A much more probable cause of tidal waves occurring at the same time in the Pacific and Atlantic would be the proximity of a large meteor or asteroid. Was there such an occasion? Yes! The German scientist and inventor Otto Muck in *The Secret of Atlantis*, states that a possible cause of the sinking of Poseidonis was an asteroid, which struck the Earth. Referring to modern times, he also gave the date when the asteroid Adonis, six miles in diameter, deviated from its orbit, came within 186,000 miles of the Earth, and was almost captured by it. "We can only feel immense gratitude for our lucky escape from a horrible danger," says Muck. The date of this event? Muck gives it as February 1936.

Another accomplishment was that all discarnates (the earth-bound souls, in between embodiments, hovering in the Earth's atmosphere) over Southern California were removed, and led into higher realms. One of the most vicious ancient vortexes of destructive force was removed from the city of San Pedro, west of Long Beach. One-third of the destructive accumulation of mankind was dissolved and removed from the Earth forever.

Never was there ever anything written in the entire history of mankind as important as the book *I AM Discourses* (dictations by the Ascended Master Saint Germain). The Ascended Master Jesus commented on this book as follows; "Stand 100% in and with your *I AM Discourses* and you will have such freedom, such joy, such accomplishment that will forever dissolve all doubt and fear from your consciousness."

Twenty thousand healings were attributed to Mr. Ballard. According to the "eyewitness," many people were healed while attending the lectures and hearing the messages given by the Masters through Mr. Ballard.

Saint Germain summarized the accomplishments of 1934 to 1939 best when He said; "The great achievements of these five years through these humble messengers and your (the student body) wonderful assistance are unparalleled in the history of the earth."

References to World Wars I & II

The Masters provided some interesting comments on World War I and World War II.

Apparently Kaiser Wilhelm (of W.W.I.) and Hitler were under the influence of a black magician who lived in the Black Forest. One Master stated "Do you understand why the Kaiser was and why Hitler today is in this condition? You were told last night about the last black magician who was seized and taken from the earth, and who had been anchored in the Black Forest of Germany . . . An associate of that black magician was anchored in Siberia. Many wonder why so many magnificent people were sent to Siberia, even in the time of the Czar. Those two black magicians were the most powerful in connection with the forces of the earth, but now they are no more . . ."

"The same force has hold of Mussolini and Stalin, only with Stalin it is a wholly different thing. He does not think so much of the conquest of America; but he has become wholly a fiend of destruction. He thinks of scarcely anything else in his suspicion but to destroy those of whom he is afraid, and whom he thinks might take his place. He has murdered thousands and thousands of magnificent men in Russia, because of that fiendish suspicion and dread for his own safety . . "

"Stalin is so afraid, he is afraid to sleep." (Eriel September 1939)

"You will find that these three dictators (Hitler, Mussolini and Stalin), all three of them in Europe, will suddenly collapse like a balloon." (Saint

Germain April 4, 1939)

"Only a few individuals know the real cause of W.W.I., and no doubt it is for the best." (Mr. Ballard, after being shown certain events of the Cosmic Screen by Saint Germain when visiting the Royal Teton Retreat)

"It is the absolute determination of certain people in Washington to throw America into war within six months, or after the first of the year." (Saint Germain November 26, 1939)

"We have been in Germany, Russia, France, England and some other countries. Seeing the poison that has been spread in the feeling world of these young people, really it is something that would almost wrench the heart, even that of an Ascended Being. We see the magnificent youth of those countries, whose minds are poisoned by this false pretense of the solutions to the problems of the world. It is just drawing them into the meshes of a venomous thing which will one day be their destruction. Europe stands today in the most dangerous position she has ever stood in, in her history." (given in 1938)

"Mankind today is in the greatest need in thousands of years. Unless divine assistance is given, mankind will perish under the conditions which are sweeping Europe today." (Archangel Michael November 15, 1938)

"Only a few individuals of the heads of the governments of Italy, Germany, and Russia desire destructive things. Hundreds of thousands of those blessed people are as fine as you are, but fear holds them trembling and bound." (An Ascended Being referring to W.W.II.)

"Much in Germany has been destroyed of which you do not know, but I still have the hope that the people of Germany, before it is too late, will rise, reestablish and sustain the power and love of the Christ." (Jesus, November 1939)

Mr. Ballard's Transition

In April of 1936 Mr. Ballard had qualified for his ascension. He decided to continue with this instruction to help Saint Germain bring in the Golden Age. Mr. Ballard transitioned on the last day of 1939. He had lectured to the very end.

Mr. Ballard ascended under a special dispensation obtained through the efforts of the Goddess of Light, the Goddess of Liberty, and the Ascended Being known as Mighty Victory. Under that dispensation, which applies to all mankind, it is no longer necessary for qualified lifestreams to raise the purified physical body into the Christ-Self, and then ascend into the I AM Presence, as Jesus did. The new action is that the purified essence of the physical body will be drawn into the etheric body and following this, the ascension into the I AM Presence takes place. Under the new action the outer structure, the physical form remains. This makes it much easier to gain the ascension. Saint Germain called this act of mercy the greatest gift ever offered mankind.

THE SECOND "NEW AGE" DISPENSATION

Just prior to 1952, Master El Morya contacted Master Saint Germain and asked Him to support a plan whereby El Morya would assist Saint Germain's efforts in bringing in the New Age. Saint Germain agreed. Together they went before the Solar Lords Helios and Vesta, and submitted the plan for their approval. The main reasons for the new endeavor as given by the Master El Morya were as follows:

1) The interest and enthusiasm of many students for Saint Germain's past effort had been gradually diminished. Only smoldering embers remained of a once

hopeful flame.

2) El Morya reasoned that a well-meaning student cannot consciously cooperate with the Ascended Masters unless he knows what they are doing. If given that opportunity, he will have a choice, where before he had none. Intuition is fine, but it is insufficient for billions of lifestreams stumbling through the blind mazes of human creation.

3) The spiritual Hierarchy meets twelve times a year at different Retreats. As part of this gathering, a certain amount of radiation is given to the people of the Earth. Mankind, not knowing of these events, does not respond and offer energy in return. Consequently, the Masters are prohibited by Cosmic Law to continue this effort beyond a certain point. There was a great need to acquaint students with the knowledge as to which retreat would be open during a particular 30-day cycle and to have the students return the energy sent by the Masters.

4) After the transition of Mr. Ballard, some of the dictations and publications of Saint Germain's dispensation were no longer freely available. None of the material was ever translated by Mr. Ballard's successors. This was done against the wishes of Master Saint Germain, who had urged repeatedly to have these publications distributed on a basis as wide as possible.

5) Thanks to the effort of the student body, more than the original amount of energy available to the Masters in 1934 was available in 1950. This could be used for a new effort.

6) One Master stated: "How can a Hierarchy direct the progress of the race unless it can reach the consciousness and outer mind of the lifestreams who are in distress, unless there is a bridge, a link, a connection over which Our counsel may reach the intellect of the personal self." (Reference to the need of monthly magazine intended to receive wide-spread dis-

tribution.)

7) There were additional students who had worked with El Morya in previous embodiments. These could be given an opportunity for service.

8) The Cosmic Law allowed the Earth only a limited time to prepare for the inbreath. The same held true for every planet in the galaxy, including the planet Venus. As part of this cosmic step, Sanat Kumara had to be released back to Venus within a 20-year period. This situation required emergency measures. The counsel held 100 years ago was no longer pertinent to the endeavor which engaged the energies of the Brotherhood at that hour.

9) El Morya argued that a cosmic service was required that would cover the entire planet. In this way, the current crisis could be brought under control. This cosmic service would not be completed until every individual would achieve the ascension. It included:

a) preparation of a new messenger, through which El Morya's plan could be brought to the consciousness of the people.

b) creation of a monthly magazine that would be utilized to publish His instructions and that of other Ascended Masters. This instruction would receive the widest possible circulation.

c) contact by letter to certain students that El Morya had association with in former lifetimes.

Helios and Vesta, after listening to the plan of El Morya, gave Him a limited dispensation. They stated that He should seek the consent of Sanat Kumara, the Maha Chohan, and the Karmic Board, and that a permanent dispensation could only be granted if there were sufficient response from the students contacted by letter.

After returning from Helios and Vesta, El Morya contacted the aforementioned Beings of the Hierarchy of the Earth. They acquiesced to the plan, the Maha

Chohan asking El Morya if He had forgotten His experience with the Theosophical Society and reminding him He would have to replenish the cosmic stockpile of energy himself, if there was inadequate response from the students. El Morya agreed to this condition, and said He would like to go ahead and try. El Morya added that he would like to prove to the Karmic Board, that mankind, once enlightened, would serve and unite for the common purpose of releasing Sanat Kumara so He could return to Venus.

Then El Morya wrote several letters to a few students, asking them to actively support His effort. Not all of them agreed to do so, but the response was sufficient to obtain a permanent dispensation.

El Morya was able to obtain the support of Geraldine Innocente, His unascended twin-flame. She became the new messenger. According to the "eyewitness", Geraldine had been embodied several times as an oracle of Delphi. The Masters were able to use Geraldine as a channel by accelerating the vibrations of her mental and emotional bodies, and by using the brain consciousness and the vocal cords for reception.

Frank C. Pita and Mrs. Francis Ekey volunteered to become the manager and associate editor of the monthly journal of "The Bridge to Freedom." Its first publication occurred in April 1952. Geraldine's mother helped also; she wrote articles in the journal under the pen name "T.D. Marches." El Morya became the editor of the journal, using the name "Thomas Printz." According to El Morya, he chose the name Thomas from His former embodiment as Thomas Moore. So "Thomas prints" became Thomas Printz.

El Morya had hoped to bring the new activity in as a supplement to Saint Germain's ongoing effort under the "I AM Activity." Until the end He had hoped to obtain Mrs. Ballard's support, or at least to avoid her active opposition. She appeared before the "Bridge to Freedom" group in Philadelphia, declaring she was the only authorized messenger, (source: "eyewitness").

Also the part of the plan asking the support of the Theosophical Society, the Rosicrucian Order, the First Church of Christ, Scientist (Christian Science), and Unity School of Christianity was unsuccessful. Under this concept each organization would have kept its identity and the basis of each group's specialized activity would have been published in the journal of the "Bridge to Freedom." Several letters were written, and excerpts of these are given for the perusal of the student. Upon being questioned on that subject, the "eyewitness" said she believed this part of El Morya's effort was partially unsuccessful because some of the leaders of those organizations would not let go of "their" students.

Following are excerpts from one dictation and several letters by Ascended Masters to various individuals and organizations, attempting to enlist their support. These are listed here because they illustrate better than anything else the goals and objectives of the new activity, called "Bridge to Freedom," as perceived by the Masters. These letters are of profound significance; they apply to our present situation as well.

Dictations by Saint Germain, September 30 and August 25, 1953:

"The endeavor of the Great White Brotherhood is to unfold the spiritual nature within every lifestream, which must be developed from within the soul of every man. Earth's children must of themselves provide the Light which is required to insure the Earth a permanent place in this solar system. This Light comes through the hearts of men. If they are not given an opportunity to learn the Law, and are denied by language restrictions and by limitations of distribution the tremendous accumulated store of wisdom that lies unprinted, how can they be counted upon to contribute their Light?

"It was for the purpose of reaching these millions that this endeavor was started, not as a new activity, but as a complement to the former, a supplement, not a competitor."

Saint Germain, in a letter to a chela, October 1, 1952

"It is to be regretted that in the *final hour* of mankind's greatest trial, the very few lifestreams who are cognizant of the Divine Plan, the Presence of God, and the Great White Brotherhood, must 'strain at the gnat and swallow the camel'.

"It was never intended to start a 'new' activity, but to broaden the field of service of the present activity, by engaging the competent and willing services of lifestreams not presently allowed full expression of their talents in 'widening the borders of the Father's kingdom.' Many hundreds of thousands of souls have not been privileged to receive the instruction brought forth in My name, due to barriers of language, limitation in the production and distribution of illuminating literature, and the unhappy 'excommunications' which resulted from misunderstandings of a human nature.

"Meanwhile, the Cosmic Law had given the Brotherhood approximately 20 years to secure the self-conscious illumination of the Earth's atmosphere, which alone could be accomplished through the expansion of the Light in the hearts of all men, the 3 1/2 billion who were presently embodied, and the 5 to 6 billion awaiting embodiment. A way and means by which We might reach the consciousness of the people had to be devised. The journal of the "Bridge to Freedom" was the solution to this problem. Mrs. Ballard was informed prior to any other individual of the purpose for which the monthly journal came forth, and was courteously invited to allow Us the opportunity of supporting her work and performing through other well-qualified individuals the task of reaching lifestreams other than those presently blessed by the knowledge of the "I AM" Activity. We shall continue to expand the workable knowledge of the Cosmic Law, and time and harvest will confirm the God intent behind this endeavor.

"The Sun cannot limit its shining to *one beam*, nor the Love of God to one human consciousness, no matter how well attuned it may have been to the vibrations of the Masters."

Letter, El Morya to Mrs. Ballard, April 1, 1952

"As the accredited messenger of the Master Saint Germain, it falls upon your shoulders to lead the people in the way of the Masters Whom you serve. The outpouring of Truth that has come forth through your consciousness and that of our beloved Brother, Mr. Ballard, is the apex of spiritual revelation in this age. The spiritual leaders of the race must unify their energies, and it is appalling that the limited consciousness of the orthodox world has preceded the awakened consciousness of the pioneers of the race in this regard. It is only the fear born of young movements that holds the leaders of the higher thought from practicing the tenets of brotherhood. The older religious orders, confident in their centuries of sworn allegiance by the greater masses of the human race, need not fear that unity means oblivion of individuality.

"While you have done well, and it was necessary to keep pure, undefiled, and uncontaminated, the revelations of the Masters of Wisdom that form the foundation of the 'I AM' Activity today, there are sheep in 'other folds,' and a collective, tolerant, active world Brotherhood, can and will be effected.

"This publication [the journal] is an esoteric magazine, solely for those who have accepted the Masters' Authority, which will act as a necessary link between the peoples of Central, South and North America, and which will render the service which your diversified activities will not allow you to perform, keeping an active, current knowledge of the work of the Brotherhood before the people, in order that all may avail themselves of the tremendous blessings that are being poured out at inner levels. Conscious knowledge of these activities will enable the earnest students to participate actively in the Hierarchy's Cosmic Work.

"The proposed spiritual digest will be an esoteric release, combining the best fruits of all present day thought on a spiritual line, but the undercurrent will hold fast to the principles upon which Saint Germain's Activity was founded, and will gently lead the people into the understanding that is found within the Cosmic Messages of that publication and the active participation of the lifestream on Earth in drawing and focusing the necessary energies to make the golden Age of Freedom a fact, and not an ephemeral dream."

Master Serapis Bey to Mrs. Ballard written just prior to April, 1952

"Some time ago you stood before me and asked for help for the American people. The time has come when I may stretch forth My hand and proffer that assistance. Although you have accomplished so much, yet the time alloted by the Cosmic Law for the balancing of the Earth's account is running out. Venus must move onward in its journey toward the Sun. Sanat Kumara must of necessity be with His planet during this initiation. We, of Earth, must 'loose Him' and let him go. We can only accomplish this by providing His successor and by generating enough Light within the Earth to meet the Cosmic Law's demand. Much remains to be done. Through the medium of the (Bridge) Journal, which We have prepared, We will endeavor to fill in the services which one small body, no matter how willing, cannot render. Main among them will be:

1. Widen the scope of Truth's message to include all the peoples in the Western Hemisphere, which is to be the stage of the final drama of Earth's experience.
2. Acquaint the interested peoples in the current important activities taking place in the Retreats and Council Halls of the Hierarchy while they are in progress. In this way, We can secure the cooperation of their voluntary energies in our proposed plans.
3. Create a feeling of tolerance, interest and active Brotherhood among the many units who are working toward world progress, but whose endeavors lack the strength of unified, conscious action.
4. Herd the peoples into the fold of Saint Germain's instruction, release the Cosmic message through His messenger, and encourage the active participation in the decrees by which our planet will become free.

"These are all in accord with your design. They are services of the Brotherhood that you have not had time to organize. They are motivated by the desire to promote Saint Germain's kingdom, and they are offered to you, humbly, by Those you serve, to 'widen the borders of your kingdom.'"

Letter, El Morya to the President of the Theosophical Society, August 25, 1951

"Be not like the young man in Rabindranath Tagore's poem, whose lifetime search for the magic touchstone was defeated for lack of perception, humility, and discernment.

"Man has always fashioned a 'vessel' for the Truth which he sought, and then blindly and angrily denied all Truth that did not magnetize itself through his crudely-fashioned vessel. The Jews rejected their Messiah, and those who love the Brothers best, deny Their right and power to speak unless it be through lips that they, the chelas, choose to sanctify.

"You are raised to a position of authority and responsibility to many thousands of earnest, searching souls. Be not like the Pharisees of old, for your karma is bound to the progress of the Society, and the worth of the Society lies in its active participation in the endeavors of the Brotherhood at the present time. What benefit to the race to admire and study the achievements of a generation gone? Life has progressed, human needs have changed, international appearances must be dealt with as of today.

"Think you that We, the Brotherhood of Life, are not abreast of the times? Yet if you deny Us speech and presence, how can you and the vast army of souls you lead, qualify to serve a Cause whose present daily activities are hidden behind the veil which you do not choose to lift?

"We are here. We are waiting to give you the orders of today. Oh, yes, through the clumsy instruments of 'intuition' and the finer 'perceptions,' a portion of our thought must reach the more 'elect', but, We may rend the veil and speak forth fully, freely, precisely now while We may reach the intellect of the people who have signified a desire to serve.

"Open your heart, Brother. Read of the 'fruit' and testify to the tree whose branches have been your canopy since youth. Let Our Presence flow through the works of the Society and resuscitate its early powers as an instrument in the hands of Those Who know."

Letter, El Morya to Mrs. Ballard, Theosophical Society, Christian Science, Rosicrucian Society & Unity School of Christianity, April 1, 1952

"It is time that the pioneers of the spiritual highway joined together the energies of their people to more effectually stem the tide of evil that must be rooted out of the human race before the permanent Age of Peace and world Brotherhood can be established.

"It is certainly for the spiritually elect, those whose studies and convictions have given them a clearer and deeper insight into the causes acting behind the present manifestations of world chaos than orthodox theology can offer, to put aside their separate interests and individual prides, and meet together on a common ground, presenting a united front to the small minority of misguided humanity who are responsible for the menace of communism and war. The founder of the fine organization, The Christophers, wisely points out that less than one per cent of mankind is responsible for the major distresses that beleaguer the great majority of the people. Their unpleasant strength lies in the unity of their energies, endeavors and disintegrating purpose.

"The purpose of your spiritual organization is <u>one</u> with the purpose of all other sincere organizations dedicated to enlightening mankind and leading them upon the path toward self-mastery and individual completeness. The perfecting and illuminating of each member of the human race, no matter by which road he may travel, is essential to an active, effective world Brotherhood, in which peace, opulence, health and expanding perfection may be created, sustained and consciously expanded. The old story of the 'one rotten apple in the barrel' is most assuredly applicable to the mankind of Earth.

"The greater majority of the people are 'followers' of a few God-chosen individuals to whom they look for their pattern, their course, their reception or rejection of Truth or fallacy, as the case may be. It is, therefore, up to the leaders of the metaphysical, the occult, and spiritual schools to use the prerogative of their leadership and to exercise the influence of their wisdom and judgment in helping to 'join' forces of the constructive people of the world of tolerant, understanding, active Brotherhood, whereby the spiritual energies of their people may be combined to take and hold the control of our planet and its people against the small minorities that choose to plunge us into wars, kill our youth, and cause constant anxieties and tension in the hearts of all straight-thinking, constructive, human beings.

"To do this, it is not necessary to forego your own individual teachings, creeds, codes, rules and regulations, any more than the Catholic, Protestant or Jewish congregations have lost their individual identities in uniting their strengths. They have, however, inculcated a new spirit of tolerance in their members, and strangely enough, found a common band of Truth underlying the fundamental beliefs of their separate selves. Many books have been published on the chicanery and invalidity of various movements, but none on the common good which is served by all.

"Are you not willing to join a spiritual world movement and, through an impartial publication, allow the purpose, tenets and accomplishments of your teachings to reach all the peoples on the spiritual path? Thus, tolerant understanding, broader knowledge, will enable us to blend our strengths, unite our energies and, who knows, we may find the foundation of Truth beneath all the movements to be one.

"A caravan crossing the trackless wastes is stronger when the company is many, although each may have a separate mission, an individual interest, and at the end of the journey, each may pursue a different course.

"We await your reaction and know confidently that, because you have been chosen by God to lead a portion of the people, you are primarily desirous of forwarding the Cause of world peace, world unity, individual security and planetary freedom for all mankind from the ills to which our race is presently heir.

"We hope you will be interested in joining a humanitarian world movement in which all metaphysical and spiritual groups are represented, and, through it, knit the energies of each group into a united front against evil, bigotry, intolerance, war, disease, and hatreds of every kind. Through the offices of an impartial digest We may give the basis of each group's specialized activities to the world."

Dictation, Saint Germain, 1950's

"We had hoped to the very last to secure the support, or at least to avoid the active opposition, of Mrs. Ballard, but as this has not been possible, We shall have to pass through a period of transition, during which the sheep and the goats again must choose their respective paths and then abide in the goal to which those paths will ultimately lead.

"It is to be regretted that the very Activity which I instituted at so great a cost of energies and such a great investment of Love should have again built into the inner bodies of those who responded to My Keynote, fear and superstitions that have atrophied the reasoning processes in the mental body, and energized the emotional bodies with fanatical zeal rather than God-controlled enthusiasm.

"It is so easy for energy to get away from the original purpose for which it was dedicated, especially if the channel through which that energy has been focused diverts from the original motive which became the pulsation of the release.

"The Cosmic Law has given Us 20 years in which to accomplish an almost impossible task, the purification of the inner bodies of the race, the raising of the vibratory action of the physical body, the attunement of the brain consciousness to the heart Flame, and the expansion of the Spirit of God through the souls until each aura emits Light. Although We need thousands of trained lifestreams to assist Us, We must begin with a handful, and this handful, strongly impressed with the teachings of the various channels through which they have evolved, must be re-educated individually and collectively."

Saint Germain said on July 18, 1953, the curtain had all but closed upon His previous endeavors. (A.D.K. Luk)

Step by step, El Morya implemented His plan. A monthly publication acquainted students with the Retreat of the month. A certain course of application was given, which included the dates of the 30-day cycle the Retreat was open, the name of the Hierarch of the Retreat, the type of flame the Retreat was using, the music that contained the keynote of the Retreat, and a specific application of the rhythmic breath. There was a great response from students all over the world. On the opening date of a Retreat, students applied what they had learned; for the first time, there was a joining of energies extending from both the ascended realm and from Earth. This enabled the Masters to obtain the consent of the Beings administrating Cosmic Law to give additional assistance to the Earth, giving credence to El Morya's original idea.

Once El Morya had received His final dispensation, all members of the Great White Brotherhood joined His effort. The scope of the message was enlarged. It included many details of so-called pre-history. For the first time the wishes of the Masters were followed, and some of this work was translated. One

Ascended Being described this effort as Genesis re-written. This time it was written by Ascended Beings instead of unascended beings. New groups came into being. This created new permanent forcefields, magnetic centers which drew angels closer to the Earth and which gave the Masters greater freedom in bringing forth specific instruction and radiation. Of this effort, the Masters said that the task of the Bridge will never be complete until the very last lifestream has crossed it, on the way to his ascension.

The effort by the Masters and the students was so successful, that it enabled Sanat Kumara to return to Venus as early as 1956.

Geraldine Innocente passed through the transition August 1961. After her passing, most of her channeled dictations were no longer published.

Bibliography, Part I

Ballard, G.W., Mr. and Mrs. *Voice of the I AM.* Monthly publications. Santa Fe, New Mexico, P.O. Box 1181, Saint Germain Press, 1936 through 1940

Barker, A.T. *The Mahatma Letters to A.P. Sinnett.* Wheaton, Illinois, Theosophical Publishing House, 1972

Bethards, Betty. *Atlantis.* Novato, California 94937, P.O. Box 761, Inner Light Foundation, 1976

Churchward, J. *The Second Book of the Cosmic Forces of Mu.* New York, Paperback Library, 1935

Cayce, E.E. *Cayce on Atlantis.* New York, Castle Books, 1968

King, Godfré Ray. *Unveiled Mysteries.* Sante Fe, New Mexico, P.O. Box 1181, Saint Germain Press, 1939

Luk, A.D.K. *Law of Life*, Vol. I & II. Oklahoma City 73107, 1124 N. Meta Ave., A.D.K. Luk Publications, 1959 & 1960

Luk, A.D.K. *Law of Life and Teaching by Divine Beings*, Vol. I, II & III. Same publisher, 1978

Luk, A.D.K. *Life and Teaching of Jesus and Mary.* Same publisher, 1966

Muck, O. *The Secret of Atlantis.* New York, Times Books, 1978

Printz, T. *The Seven Mighty Elohim Speak on: The Seven Steps to Precipitation.** Kings Park, New York, The Bridge to Freedom, 1955

Printz, T. *Memoirs of Beloved Mary.* Kings Park, New York, The Bridge to Freedom, 1955

Printz, T. *The Bridge to Freedom.* Monthly journal. Kings Park, New York, The Bridge to Freedom, 1952 through 1961*

Rehwinkel, A.M. *The Flood.* Saint Louis, Concordia Publishing House, 1951

Saint Germain. *I AM Discourses.* Santa Fe, New Mexico, P.O. Box 1181, Saint Germain Press, 1939

Scott-Elliot, W. *The Story of Atlantis and the Lost Lemuria.* Wheaton, Illinois 60187, P.O. Box 270, The Theosophical Publishing House, 1972

Schmidt, F. *Mitteilungen des Eremiten (Explanations of a Hermit).* Mount Shasta, California 96067, P.O. Box 466, Ascended Master Teaching Foundation, 1982

Schmidt, F. *Kundgebungen des Eremiten* (Messages a Hermit).* Cleveland, Ohio, Felix Schmidt, 1951

* No longer published

PART II
ATLANTIS VERIFIED

1 - Plato's Dialogues

INTRODUCTION

Next to the Bible, no other subject has fascinated mankind more than the subject of Atlantis. One writer estimated that a total of 20,000 books have been written to date on Atlantis.

It is the purpose of this part of the book to demonstrate to the reader the large measure of consistency between the testimony of the Ascended Masters as given here-to-fore, and Plato's dialogues, as well as the testimony of other writers, the testimony of the ocean floor, the reports of several psychics, and the legends and customs that are common to people living on both sides of the Atlantic Ocean, all this pointing to a common origin. The testimony of other writers is presented more-or-less in a condensed version, to emphasize the conclusions they reached.

The source material for this portion of the book is listed in the bibliography. A few contributions are based on my various trips to Uxmal and Chichen-Itza in Yucaton, and a trip to the Teotihuacan Valley near Mexico City.

PLATO'S ACCOUNT

Plato (427 to 347 B.C.) was one of the greatest philosophers of Western culture. He was a student of Socrates. Plato was born in Athens; his families on both sides were among the most distinguished in Athens. Plato was reported to be descended from the Athenian statesman and lawgiver, Solon. After the death of Socrates, Plato traveled to Italy and Egypt. Upon his return, he opened a school called "The Academy," in Athens. It was the first university founded in Europe, and soon became the recognized authority in the fields of scientific research, philosophy, mathematics, and law. Plato considered the founding and organization of The Academy as his greatest accomplishment. He presided over this university for the remainder of his life. Plato stressed that in order to discover the real world of ideas and forms, man must forgo the testimony of the five material senses.

Many writers consider the *Timaeus* and *Critias* of Plato the fullest and most important body of historical evidence regarding Atlantis we possess. In *Timaeus* Plato relates certain historical events of ancient Greece and Atlantis. Additional details, including the lifestyle and customs of the people living on the island of Atlantis, are given in *Critias*. What Plato says about Atlantis fills about 20 pages.

Plato uses the vehicle of a dialogue to relate details of the Atlantean Civilization. In *Timaeus*, a person named Critias (the younger) gives the origin of this account. He names as the source an old priest living in the ancient city of Sais, in Egypt. The priest told his story to Solon, the Greek lawgiver.

Solon in turn gave it to his friend and relative Dropidas, who then gave it to a person also named Critias, the grandfather of Critias the younger.

Here are presented excerpts from Plato's story, as found in *Timaeus* and *Critias*. This version of Plato's account was prepared by comparing the following books:

1) *Atlantis, the Antediluvian World*, I. Donnelly
2) *The History of Atlantis*, L. Spence
3) *The Secret of Atlantis*, D. Muck
4) *The Stones of Atlantis*, Dr. D. Zink

These authors have used different translations as their source. There are minor differences. I have added some comments; these are shown in parenthesis. In this version, ancient units of measurement were converted into miles and feet.

Background: Socrates, Hermocrates, Critias (the younger), Timaeus and a fourth person, presumably Plato himself, have come together for the purpose of philosophical debate. Socrates reminds Critias that he promised them a story which might prove acceptable for the festival of the Goddess Athena.

Critias: "Then listen, Socrates, to a strange tale, which is, however, certainly true, as Solon, who was the wisest of the seven sages, declared. He was a relative and great friend of my great-grandfather, Dropidas, as he himself says in several of his poems. Dropidas told Critias, my grandfather, who remembered, and told us of great and marvelous exploits and one in particular, that were achieved by Athens in the days of old, which, through lapse of time and in the course of generations, have vanished from memory."

Socrates: "Very good; and what is the ancient famous action of which Critias (the elder) spoke, not as a mere legend, but as a verifiable action of the Athenian State, which Solon recounted?"

Critias: "I will tell you an old story which I heard from an aged man, for Critias was at that time nearly ninety years of age, while I was about ten."

"Tell us," said the other, "the whole story, and how and from whom Solon heard this verifiable tradition."

"There is in Egypt," said Critias, "in the Delta, at the head of which the river Nile divides, a province called Sais, and the chief city of the province is also called by that name. The founder of this city is a goddess whose name in the Egyptian tongue is Neith, and in Greek, as the Egyptians say, Athena. The people of Sais are great lovers of the Athenians and claim a certain kinship with us. Now when Solon traveled to this city, he was most honourably treated by its people, and when he inquired about ancient things of the priests, who were most learned therein, he found that neither he nor any other Greek knew anything about such matters.

"Thereupon, one of the priests, who was of very great age, said, 'O Solon, Solon, you Hellenes are but children, and there is never an old man who is an Hellene.' Solon, hearing this, said, 'What do you mean?' 'I mean to say,' replied the priest, 'that in mind you are all young; there is no old opinion handed down among you by ancient tradition, nor any science. The legends preserved here are the most ancient on record. Now when in Athens or in Egypt, or in any other known place anything noble or great or otherwise notable did occur, we wrote it down and preserved an account of it from ancient times in our temple here. For, in the first place, you remember one deluge only, whereas there were many of them; and, in the next place, you do not know that there dwelt in your land the fairest and noblest race of men which ever lived, of whom you and your whole city are but a seed or remnant and this was unknown to you, because for many generations the survivors of that destruction died and made no sign.'

The priest continued, 'For there was a time, Solon, before that great deluge of all, when the city which now is Athens was first in war, and was preeminent for the excellence of her laws, and is said to have performed the noblest deeds, and to have had the fairest constitution of any of which tradition tells, under the face of heaven.' Solon marvelled at this, and earnestly requested the priest to inform him exactly and in order about these former citizens. 'You are welcome to hear about them, Solon,' said the priest, 'both for your own sake and for that of the city; and, above all, for the sake of the goddess who is the common patron and protector and educator of both our cities. She founded your city a thousand years before ours, receiving from the Earth and Hepaestus the seed of your race, and then she founded ours, the constitution of which is set down in our sacred registers as 8000 years old.

'But concerning the citizens of Athens nine thousand years ago, I will briefly inform you of their laws and of the noblest of the deeds which they performed. Many great and wonderful deeds are recorded of your state in our histories; but one of them exceeds all the rest in greatness and valor; for these histories tell of a mighty power which was aggressing wantonly against the whole of Europe and Asia, and to which your city put an end. This power came forth out of the Atlantic Ocean, for in those days the Atlantic was navigable; and there was an island situated in front of the straits which you call the Columns of Heracles [Straits of Gibraltar]: the island was larger than Libya and Asia put together, and was the way to other islands, and from the islands you might pass to the entire continent which surrounded the true ocean; for this sea which is within the Straits of Heracles is only a harbor, having a narrow entrance, but that other is a real sea, and the surrounding land may be most truly called a continent.

'On this island of Atlantis there existed a great and admirable empire, which had taken possession of the entire island as well as of the other islands and of parts of that continent; and besides these they ruled over the parts of Libya within the Columns of Heracles as far as the borders of Egypt, and over Europe as far as Tyrrhenia [The Tyrrhenian Sea is located between Sardinia and Italy, Donnelly identifies Tyrrhenia with today's Italy].

'This mighty power once tried to subdue both your country and ours and everything situated within the strait in a single attack. Then, O Solon, did the power of your city shine forth in all men's eyes, glorious in valour and strength. For, being foremost upon earth in courage and the arts of war, sometimes she was leader of the Hellenes, sometimes she stood alone perforce when the rest fell away from her; and after being brought into the uttermost perils, she vanquished the invaders and triumphed over them, and preserved from slavery those who were not yet subjected, and freely liberated all the others who dwelt within the limits of Heracles.

'But later when there came violent earthquakes and floods the entire valiant generation of your people was swallowed up by the earth, and the island of Atlantis was similarly swallowed by the sea and vanished in a single dreadful day and in a single dreadful night.

'And that is the reason why the sea in those parts is impassable and impenetrable, because there is such a quantity of shallow mud in the way; and this was caused by the subsidence of the island.'" (Plato's Dialogues, ii., 517, *Timaeus.*)

This ends the description given in *Timaeus.* The next passage in Plato's works which gives reference to Atlantis is his *Critias*, where a person by that name continues his account of Atlantis.

Critias: "Let me begin by observing, first of all, that nine thousand was the sum of years which elapsed since the war which was said to have taken place between all those who dwelt outside the Pillars of

Heracles and those who dwelt within them: this war I am now to describe. One of the combatants was the city of Athens, which ruled over many people. The other force was led by the kings of the islands of Atlantis, which, as I was saying, once had an extent greater than that of Libya and Asia.

"Many great deluges have taken place during the nine thousand years, for that is the number of years which have elapsed since the time of which I am speaking.

"And next, if I have not forgotten what I heard when I was a child, I will import to you the character and origin of their adversaries; friends should not keep their stories to themselves, but have them in common. Yet, before proceeding farther in the narrative, I ought to warn you that you must not be surprised if you should hear Hellenic names given to foreigners. I will tell you the reason for this: Solon, who was intending to use the tale for his poem, made an investigation into the meaning of the names, and found that the early Egyptians, in writing them down, had translated them into their own language. He recovered the meaning of the several names and retranslated them, and copied them out again in our language. My great-grandfather, Dropidas, had the original writing, which is still in my possession, and was carefully studied by me when I was a child. Therefore, if you hear names such as are used in this country, you must not be surprised, for I have told you the reason of them."

In the continuing of this dialogue, which lasted several days, Critias painted a vivid picture of the island of Atlantis; its incomparable lush vegetation, its inhabitants and glorious cities, especially the capital with the royal castle, and gave all the details from the accounts handed down by the Egyptians through Solon and Critias, the Elder.

"I have before remarked, in speaking of the allotments of the gods, that they distributed the whole earth into portions differing in extent, and made themselves temples, and sacrifices. And Poseidon, receiving for his lot the island of Atlantis, begat children by a mortal woman, and settled them in a part of the island which I will proceed to describe.

"A plain extended from the sea toward the center of the island; of all the plains it was said to be the most beautiful and excellent. A mountain rose, gently sloping in all directions, near this plain, but also toward the center, at a distance of 5.7 miles. One of the men that grew there from the earth at the beginning, by the name of Euenor, lived on top of it with his wife, Leucippe; they had an only daughter called Cleito. Her father and mother died when she grew up. Poseidon was attracted to Cleito and they became lovers. He fortified the mountain on which she lived by cutting it off from the island surrounding it, making alternate circles of canals and land, two of land, three of sea, around the center of the island and everywhere equidistant from each other so that the mountain they encircled was inaccessible to man, for there were no ships and navigation yet.

"Being a god, He found no difficulty in making special arrangements for the centre island, bringing two streams of water under the earth, which he caused to ascend as springs, one of warm water, and the other of cold, and making every variety of food to spring up abundantly in the earth. He also begat and brought up five sets of twins, all male, dividing the island of Atlantis into ten portions: he gave to the first-born of the eldest pair his mother's dwelling and the surrounding allotment, which was the largest and best, and made him king over the rest; the others he made princes, and gave them rule over many men and a large territory. And he named them all: the eldest, who was king, he named Atlas, and from him the whole island and the ocean received the name of Atlantic. To his twin-brother, who was born after him, and obtained as his lot the extremity of the island toward the Pillars of Heracles, as far as the country which is still called the region of Gades in that part of the world. [The Worldbook Atlas shows that the City of Cadiz, located on the southern tip of Spain, was called Gades in ancient times.]

"All these and their descendants were the inhabitants and rulers of divers islands in the open sea; and also, as has been already said, they held sway in the other direction over the country within the Pillars as far as Egypt and Tyrrhenia.

"The posterity of Atlas maintained the sovereign power during several centuries in uninterrupted succession. Their riches were so great that they surpassed those of the kings who lived in the centuries preceding their own, and no monarch of the succeeding ages could in this respect compare with them. By their wise industry they filled the capital city and the country with everything that was useful and agreeable to existence. Their power procured them all the productions of foreign lands.

"Their island furnished them with all kinds of stones and minerals, and, above all, with that mineral known as orichalcum (mountain copper) the most precious, next to gold, of all the metals. The island also produced in abundance all kinds of timber suitable for building construction. It nourished numerous herds of animals, both domestic and wild, and large numbers of elephants. These found plenty of food in the marshes, lakes and rivers, in the plains and the mountains. The soil also produced a wealth of roots, herbs, wood, gums, flowers and fruits, the sweet juice of the grape, corn, and vegetables in their season. Shady trees sheltered its happy people, and divers fruits appeased their hunger and thirst, especially one with a hard rind, affording both meat, drink and ointment. In a word, there was to be found in this island, which has so unhappily disappeared, everything which could satisfy the body and the spirit. And as they had everything provided by the land, they erected temples and royal palaces and harbors and docks and organized the rest of the country, proceeding as follows:

"Their first task was to build bridges across the rings of water surrounding the old metropolis to construct a road to and from the royal castle. They built the royal castle at the very beginning in the abode of the goddess, and their ancestors, the kings, received it from their fathers, adding as much as they could to its beauty, trying to outdo their predecessors until they had made the residence amazing to behold because of its size and beauty. For they had a canal dug 300 feet wide, a hundred feet deep, and 5.7 miles long from the sea to the outermost ring; they dug an entrance large enough to admit the largest ships; they also cut through the rings of land between the rings of water toward the bridges, wide enough for a trireme [large boats] to pass from one to the other. They roofed over the cuts so that the ships could pass underneath; for the rims of the rings were sufficiently high for this. But the largest ring of water that gave access to the sea had a width of 1800 feet; the next ring inside it was of the same width; of the two following rings the water ring was 1200 feet wide, and the ring it surrounded was just as wide. The ring of water surrounding the island's center had a width of 600 feet, but the island on which the royal castle stood had a diameter of 3000 feet. They surrounded this, as well as the rings of water, and the bridges of 100 feet width with a stone wall, with towers and gates on the bridges everywhere along the passages to the sea.

"The stone of which these immense piles were constructed was quarried from the island, and was black and red in color. The walls which encircled the outward zone were covered with a light coating of brass; those of the interior had plates of tin, and the walls of the citadel were coated with orichalcum.

"The palaces in the interior of the acropolis were constructed this way: In the centre was a holy temple dedicated to Cleito and Poseidon, which remained inaccessible, and was surrounded by an enclosure of gold; this was the spot in which they originally begat the race of the ten princes, and there they annually brought the fruits of the earth in their season from all the ten portions, and performed sacrifices to each of them. Here, too, was Poseidon's own temple, six hundred feet in length and three hundred feet in width, and of a proportionate height. All the outside of the temple, with the exception of the pinnacles, they covered with silver, and the pinnacles with gold. In the interior of the temple the roof was of ivory, adorned everywhere with gold and silver and orichalcum; all the other parts of the walls and pillars and floor they lined with orichalcum. In the temple they placed statues of gold: there was the god himself standing in a chariot — the charioteer of six winged horses — and of such a size that he touched the roof of the building with his head; around him there were one hundred Nereids riding on dolphins.

"There were many other statues, votive offerings of the citizens. The temple was ringed by gold statues of all the kings, their queens, and all the offspring of the ten kings, and by many other large votive offerings by the kings as well as by private citizens, some from the city itself, others from one of the dominions. The size and design of the altar was worthy of the entire building and the royal castle and similarly expressed the greatness of the realm and the splendor of the temple.

"In the next place, they used fountains both of cold and hot springs; these were very abundant, and both kinds wonderfully suited for use by reason of the sweetness and excellence of their waters. They constructed buildings about them, and planted suitable trees; also cisterns, some open to the heaven, others which they roofed over, to be used in winter as warm baths: there were the king's baths, and the baths of private persons, which were kept apart. There were also separate baths for women, and others again for horses and cattle, and to them they gave as much adornment as was suitable for them. The water which ran off they carried, some to the grove of Poseidon, where were growing all manner of trees of wonderful height and beauty, owing to the excellence of the soil; the remainder was conveyed by aqueducts which passed over the bridges to the outer circles.

"There were many temples built and dedicated to many gods; also gardens and places of exercise, some for men, and some set apart for horses, in both of the two islands formed by the zones; and in the centre of the larger of the two there was a race-course 600 feet in width, and in length allowed to extend all around the island. Also there were guard houses at intervals for the body-guards, the more trusted of whom had their duties appointed to them in the lesser zone, which was nearer the Acropolis; while the most trusted of all had houses given them within the Citadel.

"The wharves were full of triremes and all the appliances required for them. This is how the residence of the kings was arranged: once the three outer rings of water had been crossed, a wall was reached that began at the edge of the sea, running in a circle at a distance of 5.7 miles from the largest ring enclosing the mouth of the canal into the sea. The whole was surrounded by many densely populated houses, and the roads and the largest harbor were crowded with ships and merchants arriving from all directions and creating a multitude of voices, bustle and noise by day and by night.

"I have now told you everything about the city and everything connected with this ancient settlement as it had been described to me at the time; I must now try to recall also the natural condition of the rest of the country and its organization. To begin with, the whole region was said to be very high above and steeply rising from the sea; but the whole plain surrounding the city was in turn completely enclosed by mountains which came down to the sea; the plain was uniformly flat, oblong, measuring in length 341 miles, and in width, rising from the sea, 227 miles. This part of the island was open to the south and sheltered by mountains from the north wind. The mountains surrounding it were highly praised at the time, because their number, height, and beauty far surpassed that of those found there now, and also because they contained many populous settlements as well as rivers, lakes, and meadows that supplied all wild and domestic animals with abundant food, and vast forests that offered a great variety of trees, providing an abundance of timber for woodwork of all kinds.

"This, then, was the natural condition of the plain, which was, however, cultivated by many kings over a long time. An oblong, for the biggest part leveled, was the basic shape, and what was missing from it was added by the trench surrounding it. As for its depth, width and length, it sounds incredible that in addition to the other structures there should have been such a large, artificial one, but I must pass on what I have heard about it. It was 100 feet deep, 600 feet wide throughout and, because it had been dug around the entire plain, 1136 miles long. It collected the rivers coming down from the mountains and skirted the city on both sides, discharging them into the sea. From its upper part, straight canals, most of them a hundred feet wide, led into the plain and from there to the part of the ditch that emptied into the sea, each a distance of 11.4 miles from the next. It was thus possible not only to float timber from the mountains to the city but also to transport seasonal produce in canal craft after they had dug cross links between the canals and the city.

"Twice in the year they gathered the fruits of the earth, in winter having the benefit of the rains and in summer introducing the water of the canals. As to the population, each of the lots in the plain had an appointed chief of men who were fit for military service and the size of the lot was to be a square of 6000 feet each side, and the total number of all the lots was sixty thousand.

"The leader was also obliged to provide the sixth part of a war chariot (a total of ten thousand), two horses and riders, as well as a cart without a seat, drawn by two horses and carrying a warrior armed with a small shield, who dismounted for battle, and a charioteer, two archers, two slingers, three lightly-armed stone throwers and three lancers, and four sailors for the manning of twelve hundred warships.

"Each of the ten kings, in his own division and in his own city, had the absolute control of the citizens, and in many cases, punishing and slaying whomsoever he would.

"Now the relations of their governments to one another were regulated by the injunctions of Poseidon as the law had handed them down. These were inscribed on a column of orichalcum, which was situated in the middle of the island, at the temple of Poseidon, where the people were gathered together every fifth and sixth years alternately.

"During the gathering they consulted on affairs of common concern, investigated whether someone was guilty of any misdeed and passed judgement on him. Before they assembled in court, they exchanged mutual pledges as follows: they vowed to pronounce judgement according to the laws inscribed on the column and to punish whoever had violated any of those laws; not knowingly to transgress any of them in the future, and not to usurp the rule of the country nor to obey another ruler unless he ruled according to the laws of his father.

"Sitting on the ground in the light of the glowing embers of the sacrifice they pronounced judgement on each other at night, after all the fires had been extinguished in the shrine, on any complaints of violations of the law. They recorded the judgment they had given on a gold tablet as soon as the day had dawned, and deposited them as memorials together with their robes. There were many other laws determining the duties of each of the kings: the most important one was that they should never make war upon one another, and assist one another should any one of them in some state attempt to destroy the Royal House and that they should jointly, following the tradition of their forefathers, discuss decisions about wars and other enterprises and accord supremacy to the House of Atlas. And none of the kings should have the power of life and death over any of his kinsmen unless more than half of the ten had shown agreement.

"The power of such extent and quality that ruled in these regions was instituted in that country by the god, and for many generations, as long as the nature of the god was active in them, they obeyed the laws and loved their divine kinsman. For their feelings were sincere and generous, in that they practiced gentleness and consideration during misfortune and toward one another.

"They despised everything but virtue, not caring for their present state of life, and thinking lightly on the possession of gold and other property, which seemed only a burden to them; neither were they intoxicated by luxury; nor did wealth deprive them of their self-control; but they were sober, and saw clearly that all these goods are increased by virtuous friendship with one another, and that by excessive zeal for them, and honor of them, the good of them is lost, and friendship perishes with them.

"By such reflections, and by the continuance in them

of a divine nature, all that which we have described grew and increased in them; but when this divine portion began to fade away in them, and became diluted too often, and with too much of the mortal admixture, the human nature got the upper-hand, then, they being unable to bear their fortune, became unseemly, and to him who had an eye to see, they began to appear as of a base and lower nature and had lost the fairest of their precious gifts; but to those who had no eye to see the true happiness, they still appeared glorious and blessed at the very time when they were filled with unrighteous power. Zeus, the god of gods, who rules with law, and is able to see such things, perceiving that an honorable race was in a most wretched state, and wanting to inflict punishment on them, that they might be chastened and improved, called all the gods into his most holy habitation, which, being placed in the centre of the world, sees all things. And when he had called them together he spake as follows:" (Here Plato's story abruptly ends and some believe, so-called death interfered, preventing Plato from finishing his account.)

PLATO'S ACCOUNT ANALYSED

Plato and Solon

Plato gives a scientifically-detailed description that is internally consistent and can be checked. Unlike myths and legends, including that of some of the Biblical patriarchs, there is for Atlantis as solid an evidence as there is for other items of prehistory. The evidence goes a long way to prove that Plato was an objective chronicler. He describes an educated, cultured, and relatively wealthy people. Many parts of Plato's story can be paralleled with descriptions of ancient Egypt and Peru; in fact, in some respect, his account falls short of the description of the grandeur attributed to these countries, as given by Herodotus and Prescott.

Plutarch's *Life of Solon* is the beginning of the historically-verified Greek Atlantis tradition. It is better documented than many other facts that have been accepted by official historical research.

According to Plutarch, between 571 B.C. and 562 B.C. Solon traveled to Egypt, and his first destination was Sais and Heliopolis. Here he was told by Sonchis, a priest at Sais and Psenophis, and a priest at Heliopolis, that 9,000 years ago the relations of the Egyptians with the lands to the west had been interrupted, and mud had made the sea impassable after the destruction of Atlantis by earthquakes. Solon then continued his travels and visited Cyprus. Here he was received by king Philocyprus. In honor of Solon's accomplishment, a city on Cyprus, called Aepee, was changed to Soloi.

The philosopher, Proclus (A.D. 412-485), tells us that 300 years after Solon's voyage to Egypt, that is about 260 B.C., a Greek by the name of Crantor came to Sais and saw there at the temple of Neith a column, completely covered with hieroglyphs, on which the history of Atlantis was recorded. Scholars translated the hieroglyphs for Crantor and he testified that their translation fully agreed with Plato's account of Atlantis. Is this priceless column, still hidden and preserved in the silt of the Nile, awaiting its discovery?

Some discredit Plato, stating that Plato fabricated the *Timaeus* and *Critias* to further his personal ambitions. I believe such a view is absurd. Why would a person belonging to one of the most distinguished families of Athens, serving as the president of the Academy, a most prestigious university, choose the occasion of the Festival of the Goddess of Truth, and in the presence of his beloved teacher, Socrates, tell a fairy tale? Why would he bring potential disrespect to Socrates, Critias, Dropidas and Solon, all of which have a place in history? According to Plato's dialogue, Socrates himself believed the account of the priest at Sais, because he says "[it] is not a mere legend, but a verifiable action . . . which Solon recounted."

Location and Size of Atlantis

Let us examine Plato's statements concerning the geographical location of Atlantis, its size and the extent of its empire.

It seems reasonable to state that if there is written testimony concerning a civilization of the remote past, then this record refers to the last stage of that civilization, not the initial one.

If we assume the dictations of the Ascended Masters as truthful and correct, then Plato's "Atlantis" is really its remaining fragment, which the Masters called Poseidonis. Helen Blavatsky says the same. In her book *Secret Doctrine* she states that Plato's account refers to Poseidonis.

Blavatsky called Plato an initiate. The Rosicrucion Order says something similar. Plato is identified an initiate of an early mystery school. If Plato was indeed an initiate, then it would have been his solemn duty to partially veil the truth contained in his record. We can readily see that this was done. The record was presented in the form of an allegory, a play.

With regards to the location of Poseidonis, there

hardly can be any doubt, namely, the island was located within the Atlantic Ocean. Plato's description is very clear on this point. Most or all of the ancient writers agree that the Columns of Heracles, sometimes called Columns of Hercules, are identical with today's Straits of Gibraltar. The description referring to the "true ocean" as compared to a "harbor," namely to the much smaller Mediterranean Sea, and the reference to the American Continent as surrounding the true Ocean, is so clear it should not need any additional comment.

Plato stated the island (Poseidonis) was larger than Libya and Asia put together.

Ancient historians called the region known today as Asia Minor, Asia. A map prepared by Herodotus (484 to 424 B.C.) showed the then-known area of the world in a circular-shaped map. The Mediterranean is shown in the center, to the north of it a portion of Europe is depicted, then we can notice a portion of North Africa including Libya, and finally a portion of Asia, namely today's Asia Minor. According to Otto Muck, a German engineer, holder of 2000 patents and author of *Secrets of Atlantis*, Herodotus' map resembles an older map by the Chaldeans.

What did early historians think about the subject of Atlantis?

Aelian in his *Varia Historia* states that the Greek historian Theopompus (400 B.C.) recorded an interview between King Midas and Silenus, in which the latter referred to the existence of a continent beyond the boundaries of Europe, Libya and Asia.

Strabo, a historian of about 50 B.C., mentions in his *Second Book* that a man called Poseidonius stated in about 150 B.C., that as the land was known to have changed in elevation, the account of Plato ought not be regarded as fiction, and that such a continent of Atlantis might well have existed and disappeared.

Pomponius Mela, a historian of 80 A.D., expressly

affirmed in his book that Atlantis existed.

Diodorus Siculus, a historian who lived during the time of Julius Caesar, related that the Phoenicians discovered a large island in the Atlantean Ocean, beyond the pillars of Herculus, several days sail from the coast of Africa. "The island abounded in all manner of riches. The soil was very fertile, there were rivers, mountains and forests. Fish and game were in great abundance, the climate was mild, and the trees bore fruit all seasons of the year. It was the custom of the people to retire during the summer to magnificent country homes which stood in the midst of beautiful gardens."

According to Spence, the ancient City of Carthage, near the Mediterranean Sea, was laid out in a pattern similar to the Royal City described by Plato. Carthage had a citadel hill encircled by zones of water and land, a canal to the sea, and bridges across the canals separating the land zones. There was a sea wall, guarding the entrance to the harbor.

Scott-Elliot in his book, *Atlantis and the Lost Continent of Lemuria*, describes the layout of a major coastal city that existed in the early days of Atlantis. He also calls it "Royal City." Scott-Elliot shows it to be at a location much to the south of Plato's Atlantis. The description of the layout of this city matches Plato's Royal City in almost every category.

Ignatius Donnelly, a former U.S. congressman for eight years, and author of the book, *Atlantis, the Antediluvian World*, concludes that the description contained in Plato's narrative about the surrounding mountains which sheltered the plain from the north, refers to the present towering peaks of the Azores. Considering that today's Pico mountain is 17,600 feet high, before the sinking of Poseidonis these peaks must have been truly majestic, and Plato's account of the mountains of a height not found today appears plausible.

Donnelly, Scott-Elliot, Muck, Spence, and Doctor Paul Schliemann, grandson of the discoverer of Troy, all place Poseidonis at or near the Dolphin's Ridge, and use the Azores as an easterly boundary.

Books published in Central America, later translated by De Bourbourg, state that a part of the American Continent originally extended far into the Atlantic Ocean. The books mention that the portion extending into the ocean was destroyed as a result of three major catastrophes.

According to Ixlilxochitl, the ancestors of the Toltecs in Mexico occupied the world in the third age; they came from the East in ships or barks. Robert Stacy-Judd, author of *Atlantis, Mother of Empires*, believes the Mayas were direct descendents of the Atlanteans.

Proclus quotes the writer Marcellus, who referred to the islands in the sea beyond the Straits of Gibraltar, saying that the inhabitants of one of the islands had learned from their ancestors about the existence of an extremely large island called Atlantis, which long ruled over all of the islands of the Atlantic.

Plato said that there was a great empire that wantonly warred against the whole of Europe, and that it dominated North Africa as far east as Egypt, and Europe as far east as Italy. In addition, Poseidonis ruled over parts of the continent that surrounded the true ocean. Its power made it possible to procure its needs from its colonies.

These statements show the power of Poseidonis over other countries. It brings to mind one of the statements in another part of this book about Mr. Ballard's trip in a blimp from Atlantis to the Yellowstone mines, during a former embodiment.

Donnelly believes that the parts of America referred to by Plato are Central America, Peru and the valley of the Mississippi, occupied by the "Mound Builders."

Muck shows Poseidonis' dominance over the eastern part of the United States, Central America and portions of South America, namely the Amazon region and Peru.

Natural Resources

Plato describes buildings of white, red and black stone on Atlantis. Black lava rocks and red and white rocks can today be found at the Azores. The same is the case with Plato's description of hot springs. Hot springs abound in the Azores.

Plato speaks of an abundant use of orichalcum (mountain copper). He describes a pillar of orichalcum at the Temple of Poseidon. At the end of the 19th century at Coligny, France, a pillar of orichalcum was discovered, such as that which stood in the Temple of Poseidon. (*The History of Atlantis*, by Lewis Spence.)

Army

In Britain and France the earliest historical accounts tell of a country broken up into cantons, ruled by kings, having a system of military service which prescribed the rules under which footsoldiers, charioteers, and slingers were recruited precisely as given by Plato, (Spence). Based on the details that Plato gives on the organization of the Atlantean armed forces and the large plain in the south of the islands, Muck estimates there were approximately one million men under arms, with a total population of 40 to 60 million.

Worship of God Poseidon

Plato did not invent the name Poseidon. The worship of Poseidon was universal in the earliest ages of Europe. (Baldwin, *Prehistoric Nations*, p. 148.)

Herodotus tells us the Greeks received their knowledge of Poseidon from the Libyans, who had always honored him. Dr. Badichon refers to the fact that during Roman times the inhabitants of North West Africa were known as Atlanteans. They made known their worship of Neptune to the Egyptians. According to many writers, Neptune and Poseidonis are the same individuals.

The early races of both hemispheres worshipped one God and believed in re-embodiment. Sun worship prevailed among the Cro-Magnons, Accads, Egyptians, Basques, Peruvians, Panamanians, American Indians, Toltecs, Aztecs and Mayas — in other words, on both sides of the Atlantic Ocean.

The religion of the Atlanteans, as Plato tells us, was pure and simple; they made no sacrifices other than fruits and flowers; they worshipped the sun as the giver of all life. In Peru a single deity was worshipped, and the Sun was honored as His representative. Quetzalcoatl condemned all sacrifices but that of fruits and flowers. Such was the case originally in Egypt; all of its temples were erected in honor of the sun, which was called "Ra." Thus, they worshipped only one God. In Peru the festival of the Sun was called Ra-mi.

Diodorus Siculus gives us another account of the Atlanteans. He states that the genealogy of their gods does not differ much from that of the Greeks. He continues, stating that the Atlanteans inhabited a rich country bordering upon the ocean, and were noted for their hospitality to strangers. They boasted that the Gods were born among them, and asserted that Uranus was their first king, that he civilized the people, and caused them to dwell in cities and to till the soil. He had under his dominion the greatest part of the world, especially that toward the west and the north. Uranus′ children were Atlas and Saturn. Atlas was the first to discover the knowledge of the sphere, whence arose the legend that he bore the world upon his shoulders.

Date of the Cataclysm

Plato states that an Egyptian priest told Solon that the destruction of Atlantis occurred 9000 years before that time, therefore about 9,600 years before Christ. In the *Mahatma Letters to A.P. Sinnett* the Master Kuthumi states, "that date (given by Plato) was not a fancy date, since the Egyptians had for millenniums preserved most carefully their records. They spoke only of Poseidonis, and would not reveal even to the great Greek legislator their secret chronology." In letter 23B Kuthumi assigned the date of 9564 B.C. to the Poseidonis cataclysm. Scott-Elliot also uses this date. The *Mahatma Letters* are stored at the British Museum in London. Kuthumi also states, as quoted in the same book, "the corroboration of tradition and history brought forward by Donnelly I find in the main as correct."

Spence gives the following dates for the different cataclysms that eventually destroyed all of Atlantis, namely 20,000 B.C., 14,000 B.C., and 10,000 B.C..

Many geologists feel there is a relationship between magnetic polar shifts and major natural catastrophes.

Hapgod subscribes to this theory, and made a detailed study of this subject. He said that periods of major geomagnetic pole shifts took place during the periods:

1) 78,000 B.C. to 73,000 B.C.
2) 53,000 B.C. to 48,000 B.C.
3) at 28,000 B.C.
4) 15,000 B.C. to 10,000 B.C.

Dr. Zink shows the date of a reversal of the Earth's magnetic field to be 10,376 B.C.. The latter is called the "Gothenburg Magnetic Flip."

Professor Emiliani identified an ancient flood occurring at 9,600 B.C., based on the growth rate of Foraminifera, a marine microorganism found in ocean sediments.

Egypt's Heritage

Egyptian priests told Herodotus that their written history dated back to 12,000 B.C.. Herodotus provides additional information. He states that the civilization of Egypt was initially of a higher state of accomplishment than at any later date, thus testifying to Egyptian ancient heritage.

James Churchward, in *The Second Book of the Cosmic Forces of Mu*, tells us that Sais was the first city built in Egypt, and that it was built by Thoth 14,000 years ago, after he had fled from King Chronos of Atlantis. Egyptians boasted that their ancestors in the lands of the West were the oldest among men on the Earth (Le Plongeon).

In 1912, Heinrich Schlieman's grandson, Dr. Schlieman, published an article about an inheritance he claimed to have received from his famous grandfather. He said he was given a bronze bowl which bore the Phoenician inscription, "from King Chronos of Atlantis." Paul also cited two papyrus rolls which his grandfather discovered in the museum at Petersburg, which suggested that Egypt had been a colony of Atlantis. One of the papyrus rolls, written by Manetho, the Egyptian priest-historian, gives reference to a period of 13,900 years as the reign of the Sages (kings) of Atlantis. This papyrus places the height of the civilization of Atlantis at the beginning of Egyptian history, approximately 16,000 years ago. Paul Schlieman mentioned the Lion Gate of Mycenae (Crete), on which an inscription was said to have been found which indicated that the first Temple of Sais was built by Misor, the ancestor of all Egyptians, and grandson of an Atlantean priest who had fled from King Chronos to the banks of the Nile, with the king's beautiful daughter.

Manetho, the Egyptian priest-historian, tells us that Egypt changed its calendric system about 11,000 years ago. Was this done in recognition of the start of a new era of accomplishment, recognizing the influence of Atlantean emigrants, just prior to the sinking of Poseidonis?

According to Donnelly, the Egyptians were the only people of antiquity who were well informed as to the history of Atlantis. The Egyptians are not known to have been a maritime people. Therefore, it is unlikely that they sent ships to Atlantis. Also there is no evidence that the Egyptian civilization was developed in Egypt itself. From this it appears very likely that the Atlanteans brought that knowledge to Egypt.

A Sudden Catastrophe?

Some have questioned Plato's statement that Poseidonis was destroyed suddenly in one dreadful night and day. In support of the argument of the possibility of a sudden catastrophe, the following items are presented:

1) During the 1775 earthquake at Lisbon, 60,000 people perished in six minutes. Many people were caught in a whirlpool, which caused the sinking of the land to about 600 feet below the surface of the water. According to Humboldt, a portion of the earth's surface four times as large as Europe was shaken at the same time. The earthquake extended from the Baltic Sea to the West Indies and from Canada to Algiers. Near Morocco the ground opened up and swallowed a village of 10,000 people, after which it closed above them.

2) In 1815 a large section of the island of Sundawa, 200 miles from Java, was devastated by volcanic eruptions and a whirlwind. The sound of the explosions was heard for 1,000 miles. Almost all of the 12,000 people of the province lost their lives; there were only 26 survivors. The whirlwind carried men, horses, and cattle in the air. Ashes darkened the sky, and floating cinders, two feet thick, extended for miles, making it difficult for ships to pass (Raffle, *History of Java*).

3) In 1819 the village of Sindree, on the eastern arm of the Indus, was submerged by an earthquake, together with an area of 2,000 square miles (Donnelly).

4) The entire coastline of South America at one time lifted up to about 15 feet and sank down in one

hour (Professor Winchell, *The Preadamites*).

5) There is evidence that the Northeast corner of South America tilted down suddenly into the Atlantic, the Northwestern coast was hoisted upwards. This action brought the Temple of Tiahuanaco to an elevation of 12,000 feet above sea-level (Peter Tompkins).

6) The asphyxiation and freezing of several hundred thousand mammoths must have been caused rather suddenly. Some of them have been found well-preserved in Northern Siberia and it is believed the catastrophe came so quickly, that some animals were caught in the act of eating.

7) Ancient records held by the Asiatic Society of Calcutta, India, frequently refer to Atlantis. In volume 8 of the *Asiatic Researches*, page 286, it reads, "Atlantis was overwhelmed by a flood." These ancient records also show that the Mahometans rushed into Egypt, burning all historical records and books of service.

8) In the *Popul Vuh*, sacred book of the Quiche Indian, Huracan, the god of terror floods the Earth. At the same time a huge conflagation is seen in the sky.

9) The *Voluspa* is an epic dating back far beyond pre-Germanic times. It was still sung in Iceland in the Middle Ages. The introductory verse states that it pertains to the most ancient history of man. The *Voluspa* points to a celestial pole shift. The Earth is found wobbling and trembling; the sun, moon and stars do not seem to know their places.

10) In a Greek myth, Paethon, who Homer tells us is another name for Helios, is unable to control the sun-chariot. It leaves its pre-scribed path and scorches half of the Earth.

11) The book of *Chilam Balams* was written in the Maya language, but is in Roman script. We can extract the following statement: "This happened

when the Earth began to awake. A fiery rain fell, rocks and trees crashed to the ground . . . And the Great Snake was torn from the sky . . . and skin and pieces of its bones fell unto the Earth . . . and arrows struck orphans and old men, widowers and widows who were alive, yet did not have the strength to live, and they were buried on the sandy seashore. Then the waters rose in a terrible flood. And with the Great Snake the sky fell in, and the dry land sank into the sea . . ."

Otto Muck believes that the *Popul Vuh*, and the book of *Chilam Balams* refer to an asteroid that hit Earth in the year 8498 B.C., causing the sinking of Poseidonis. As evidence that this actually happened, he recites two impact craters, about 23,000 feet in depth and having an area of 77 square miles, located near the Puerto Rico Plateau.

Muck also calls the reader´s attention to several aerial photos of North Carolina and South Carolina. The aerial camera did expose what looks like a crater field of World War I. More than 3,000 huge circular and oval depressions can be noticed, Muck says. Some depressions have the form of troughs; some of these are 1,300 feet long. They were caused when the asteroid exploded upon hitting the earth´s atmosphere. Only two large fragments remained; they hit the bottom of the ocean.

Muck reasons that the large fragments pierced the earth´s shell, causing gigantic submarine explosions, which in turn caused the eruption of volcanoes and earthquakes. Muck reasons that the action of the asteroid, which he calculates to have been 6 miles in diameter, was similar to an armor-piercing shell causing an enclosed vessel, under pressure, to explode. New vents were formed, increasing the chain of fire. The entire island of Poseidonis was caught in a fire trap. The escaping magma and the resulting depression in the interior of the earth caused the island to sink about two miles.

Moisture-bearing steam from the areas of eruption traveled eastward toward Europe, causing torrential downpours from clouds filled with black ash. The depression in the magma level had an additional impact, Muck theorizes; it caused adjacent land masses to subside or tilt towards the center. Here the account of the Masters and Peter Tompkins regarding the tilting of South America comes to mind.

Therefore, we must conclude that there is nothing improbable or impossible in the statement of Plato that Atlantis was destroyed suddenly in one dreadful night and day.

The Aftermath

According to Plato, the destruction of Atlantis filled the sea with mud, interfering with navigation. For thousands of years the ancients believed the Atlantic Ocean to be a muddy, shallow and dark sea (*Cosmos*, Volume II page 151). Herodotus, Plutarch, Scylax, and Aristotle agreed that shoal caused by the Atlantean cataclysm made shipping impossible for many centuries. Muck calculates the thickness of the mud, ash, and pumice from the eruptions as 330 feet, and says the surface of the Atlantic Ocean was covered for many years, causing interference with shipping.

2 - Other Evidence For Atlantis

ANCIENT MAYAN MANUSCRIPTS

When Cortez invaded Central America, practically all of the Mayan manuscripts were destroyed by priests of the so-called Christian Church. The Troano Manuscript and the Codex Cortesianus are examples of the very few documents which survived the onslaught.

The Troano MS, now kept at the British Museum, is considered to have been written 3,500 years ago (Scott-Elliot). It is a scroll of paper 30 feet long, folded in 8-inch folds, placed between two boards, and written for Mayan priests and noblemen.

Le Plongeon's translation of this manuscript is as follows; "In the sixth year of Can, on the eleventh Muluc of the month Zar, there occurred terrible earthquakes, which continued without intermission until the thirteenth Chuen [day]. The country of the hills of mud, the 'Land of Mu' was sacrificed. Being twice upheaved, it suddenly disappeared during the night, the basin being continually shaken by volcanic forces. Being confined, these caused the land to sink and rise several times and in various places. At last the surface gave way and the ten countries were torn asunder and scattered into fragments. Unable to withstand the force of the seismic convulsions, they sank with their 64 million inhabitants, 8060 years before the writing of this book."

In his explanations of Maya symbols, which are shown to be strikingly similar to those originating in Egypt, Le Plongeon interprets the picture of a kneeling woman as "Ma," but in the translation he switches it to "Mu." "Mu" in ancient Egyptian stands for "Mother" or "feminine principle." I believe the translation should read "Ma" or "Mother Land" or "Country of Origin." Therefore, Le Plongeon's Mu is not Lemuria, which sank much earlier. Further confirmation that we are really talking about Plato's Atlantis is seen by the fact that the Troano Manuscript speaks of ten countries.

The Codex Cortesianus, also translated by Le Plongeon, bears out a similar account. "By his strong will, Homen, God of Earthquakes, caused the earth to tremble after sunset; and during the night, Mu, the country of the hills of mud, was submerged. Mu was submerged by Homen during the night.

"The place of the dead ruler is now lifeless; it moves no more, after having twice jumped from its foundations. The king of the deep, while forcing his way out, has shaken it up and down, has killed it, has submerged it.

"Twice Mu jumped from its foundations. It was then sacrificed with fire. It burst while being shaken up and down violently by the earthquake. By kicking it, the wizard that makes all things move . . . sacrificed it that very night."

EARLY MAN IN AMERICA

More and more scientific researchers are questioning the traditional view of most of their colleagues, who insist that the North American Continent was first populated about 12,000 years ago by a migration from Asia over the Bering Strait.

On April 22, 1981, the Associated Press reported on men hunting mammoths in the Yukon. Dr. W. Irving, of the University of Toronto, told of the discovery of stone tools and broken animal bones at Crow River, thought to be 150,000 years old.

Dr. L. Leakey, in the late 1960's excavated a site at Calico Hills, California. He said he found evidence of the existence of man in America as early as 250,000 years ago. On October 27, 1980, in the "San Bernardino Sun", Dr. J. Bishop of the U.S. Geological Survey in Menlo Park set a date of 200,000 years for the same site. He used the uranium-thorium method.

Archaeologist Jeffrey Goodman based his conclusions on pollen samples found at a depth of 27 feet, and arrived at a date of 100,000 years for the Flagstaff, Arizona, site. He said this date was confirmed by visiting geologists.

Quarternary Research, in the July 1981 issue, included an article by a team of award-winning archaeologists, working with the support of the National Science Foundation. This article mentioned that sophisticated artifacts at the Hueyatlaco site in Mexico were at least 250,000 years old.

Many authors, including Donnelly and Spence, believe there is abundant proof that there was land between the New World and the Old World, because when the animals and the plants on both sides of the Atlantic are compared, one cannot help but notice their similarity. Donnelly shows the Rocky Mountains to be a dividing line. He says that an examination of the flora of the Pacific states shows that a great many trees common to Europe and the Atlantic states cannot be found west of the Rocky Mountains.

James Churchward and Le Plongeon find the Egyptian and Mayan alphabet strikingly similar. Le Plongeon states that one-third of the Maya tongue is pure Greek. Then he asks, "Who brought the dialect of Homer to America?"

The early costumes and traditions of people living in America and Europe were almost identical. Donnelly and Spence tell us they worshipped together the sun, they were instructed alike by an established priesthood, they were married by the joining of hands, there was a wedding cake cut by the bride, the bride was carried over the doorstep, they armed themselves with the same weapons, they dressed alike, they cooked in the same manner, used the same metals, believed in ghosts and fairies, listened to the same stories, played the same games, used the same musical instruments, danced the same dances, and built pyramids, obelisks and temples that were alike. All this they did, and yet the modern scientists ask us to believe there had never been any communication, trade or other ante-Columbian intercourse between these people.

If we can prove that on both sides of the Atlantic there were civilizations whose religious beliefs, arts, costumes, science and traditions were substantially identical, it is absurd to say that the peoples of the two continents evolved separately, without a common origin. Under these conditions there appears to be only one logical conclusion, namely both civilizations radiated from a common source.

THE TESTIMONY OF THE OCEAN FLOOR

The investigations of the ocean floor provide us with further tangible evidence of a former continent situated in the Atlantic Ocean.

Deep sea soundings were made by the United States' ship "Dolphin," the German frigate "Gazelle" and the British ships "Hydra", "Porcupine" and "Challenger." They mapped out the bottoms of the Atlantic prior to 1874. The result of this research was the discovery of three ridges which reach about 9000 feet above the ocean floor and in the Azores, St. Paul Rocks, Ascension and Tristan d'Acunha, penetrate the surface of the ocean.

The "Dolphin Ridge" extends from west of Great Britain to the Amazon River in South America. From there is a "Connecting Ridge" to St. Paul's and Ascension Island. From here the "Challenger Ridge" extends southward for a long distance.

The July 28, 1877 issue of *Scientific American* concludes that these ridges were once dry land because "the inequalities, the mountains and valleys of its surface, could never have been produced in accordance with any laws pertaining to the deposition of sediment, and therefore must have been carved by agencies acting above the water level."

The Officers of the "Challenger" found the explored areas covered with volcanic debris, the subsided lava and mud, that Plato tells us "made the sea impassable after the destruction of the island." A member of the

"Challenger" staff, in a lecture presented after the expedition, gave as his opinion, that there was an Atlantis.

Starke Gardner, a well known British geologist, referring to the "Dolphin" and "Challenger" ridges, asserts that a great tract of land formerly existed where the ocean is now, and that Ireland and Britain are the remains of its highest summits (*Popular Science Review*, July 1878). Donnelly believes that Plato's Atlantis is confined to the "Dolphin Ridge."

Among those geologists who uphold the Atlantean theory is Professor Edward Hull, whose investigations have led him to conclude that the Azores are the peaks of a submerged continent. He adds that based on his careful study of the soundings as recorded in the Admiralty Charts, at one time land-bridges spanned the Atlantic Ocean. He also concluded that during the existence of the Atlantean continent, there was a mountain ridge shutting off the Caribbean Sea from the Gulf of Mexico.

Muck attempted to reconstruct the outline of Atlantis. Using for his reconstruction Plato's description of the level plain in the south, and the towering mountains to the north, and the existing underwater contours, he arrived at a coastline that is outlined by the 10,000 feet contour below sea level. "It requires no great stretch of the imagination to recognize Plato's island in the resultant picture," Muck says. To the north he places today's Azores. He arrives at an island occupying about 77,000 square miles, located between 34 degrees and 24 degrees longitude and between 31 degrees and 41 degrees latitude.

Professor Askyenov, director of the Soviet Oceanology Institute, reported in April 1979 that the Soviets may have found a portion of Atlantis. His expedition found ruins and a horseshoe-shaped group of flat-topped mountains 300 to 600 feet below the surface of the ocean west of Gibraltar. He added that underwater pictures "show quite vividly a line of brick and stone walls, and fragments of wide steps."

In 1898 a cable-laying expedition was working at a depth of 1700 fathoms of water, 500 miles north of the Azores. A sample of tachylite was brought up from the ocean floor. This type of lava is always formed above water, not beneath it. It is also supposed to disintegrate in sea water in about 15,000 years. From this we may infer that within the last 15,000 years a volcano existed at this location and it was above the surface of the water (Zink).

During a 1947 Swedish oceanic expedition an examination of deep sea cores taken aboard the ship "Albatross," counted 60 fresh water species of algae. These species were located under marine sediment, approximately 12,000 feet below sea level. It was concluded that about 10,000 years ago a lake or river had existed at this location. The core was taken at a distance of 578 miles west of the coast of Africa, on the Sierra Leone Rise (Zink).

The oceanographic geologist, Dr. C. Emiliani, came to the conclusion that there was a flood 11,600 years ago. This he based on the results of some borings of marine sediments in the Bahama-Caribbean Gulf area. He also set the sea level at that time 130 feet below the existing level (Goodman).

In 1956 Dr. R. Malaise of the Riks Museum in Stockholm believed his colleague, Dr. P.W. Kolbe, had furnished proof of the sinking of the Mid-Atlantic Ridge. Dr. Kolbe found tiny shells of diatoms (small marine animals), when taking a core sample at a depth of 12,000 feet in this area. Some of the diatoms were exclusively the fresh-water type. "They could only have been deposited in the sediment when it was part of a fresh-water lake," said Dr. Malaise. He continued, "The only way that they could have been deposited in a fresh water lake would be for the present sea bottom to have been above sea level at one time."

Dr. Malaise added that he believed the Mid-Atlantic Ridge settled beneath the surface of the ocean 10,000 to 12,000 years ago. He concluded that, when the land barrier sank, the Gulf Stream reached the Arctic Ocean and the Ice Age ended.

Charles Berlitz stated that since 1968 aerial reconnaissance flights have brought to light man-made structures near the Bahamas, Cuba, Haiti, and San Domingo. Some of these structures look like pyramids. One of them, in the region of Bimini (an island in the Bahamas), measures 180 feet by 140 feet and looks like the stump of a pyramid. Near Cuba an entire complex of marine ruins waits to be explored. This is not a contradiction of Plato's account, since the Ascended Masters pointed out that in this area, near Cuba, there existed one of the earliest temples of the original Atlantean Continent.

In 1968 two pilots from the Association of Research and Enlightenment (the Cayce organization), noticed what since has been called a "temple site" in shallow water just north of Andros Island, 50 miles west of Nassau, and 150 miles east of Bimini. The archaeologist, Dr. Valentine, recognized that the stone foundation-like structure of about 60 feet by 100 feet resembled the floor plan of the Mayan Temple of the Turtles at Utmal, in Yucatan. The so-called temple is located in only six feet of water. Since then, twelve other underwater structures have been reported in the Andros area. Edgar Cayce had predicted this event, saying in 1940 that in the sunken part of Atlantis or Poseidonis a portion of a temple would be discovered under the slime of ages of seawater, near what is known as Bimini, off the coast of Florida. He added, "Poseidia [Poseidonis] will be among the first portions of Atlantis to rise again — expect it '68 and '69 — not so far away." (958-3; June 28, 1940)

In 1968 Dr. Valentine found two other structures, this time off North Bimini Island. They looked like walls, extending about 1900 feet, in a line paralleling the beach. The wall of pavement was formed by accurately placing together stones of various sizes. Some were rectangular.

The book *Atlantis, the Autobiography of a Search*, by Robert Ferro and Michael Grumley, shows some good underwater pictures. One picture shows at least eight round pillars, about 3 feet in diameter, and 3 feet to 5 feet in length. They were found by Count Turolla, off Bimini.

The researcher, Dr. David Zink, in his book *Stones of Atlantis* describes several expeditions to Bimini Island. His discoveries included the salvaging of an ancient stone building block. It was located at a depth of 20 feet and its dimensions were 12 inches square by 3 inches thick. The stone showed a perfectly square tongue and grove pattern, similar to that of a hardwood floor.

LEGENDS

In his book, *The Flood*, Professor Rehwinkel concludes that almost everywhere in the world the memory of a fearful cataclysm is being kept alive. There is almost complete agreement among the people concerning four main areas:

1) There was much destruction of human life and of all other living things by water.

2) A boat or an arc was provided as a means of escape.

3) A seed of mankind was preserved to perpetuate the human race.

4) Frequently the wickedness of man was given as the cause for the flood.

Tracy-Judd, author of the book *Atlantis, Mother of*

Empires, sees the Chaldean flood legend as almost identical to the Genesis account of the flood. The Chaldean story was written in 1700 B.C. or earlier. Prior to this was the Accadian version. Then there was the Hindu account in the Rig-Veda, similar to that of Genesis. The Iranian (Persian) account is also similar. Tracy-Judd adds that all flood legends from Asia and Europe and the Americas resemble each other. Some details of the legends are repeated here.

- The Sumerian legend states that Ut-napishtim, an ancestor of Gilgamesh and the Sumerian equivalent of Noah, describes the inundation of Mesopotomia by inky rains and tidal waves. He was the only man warned in time by the god Era. He built an ark and this way survived the catastrophe. Wolley's discovery at Ur of a layer of alluvial clay, about 8 feet thick, buried beneath 40 feet of desert sand and devoid of archaeological finds, bears out the description of the Sumerian legend (Muck).
- Brimsley le Poer Trench declared "Mythology is condensed history." Donnelly agrees, and believes the Greek gods were human beings. Based on a comparison of several legends, he reasons that the Greek god Zeus was one of the kings of Atlantis.
- The Celts believed that a part of their country once extended far into the Atlantic, and was subsequently destroyed (Donnelly).
- According to Donnelly, in the Phoenician legends, Poseidon is mentioned as the founder and king of Atlantis.
- Numez de la Vega refers to an ancient book in the Mayan tongue — how Votan (called Quetzalcoatl by the Quiche Indians) was commanded to proceed to Mexico to civilize the country. Coming to Central America, he founded the city of Palenque (Spence).
- The *Popul Vuh*, a mythological book of the ancient Maya speaks of a visit by three sons of the King of Quiches to a land in the east on the shores of the

sea where their fathers had originally come, from which they brought back, among other things, a system of writing (Bancroft, *Native Races*).

- The Nahua Family were ancestors of the Toltecs. Their leader was Quetzalcoatl. He came from the distant East and became the high priest of the Nahuas. Quetzalcoatl was a white man with a flowing beard. He wore a mitre on his head, and was dressed in a long white robe reaching to his feet. His habits were ascetic; he never married and was most chaste and pure in life. He condemned sacrifice, except for fruits and flowers, and was known as the God of peace. When somebody spoke to him about war, he placed his fingers in his ears. Quetzalcoatl invented gem-cutting and metal-casting, originated letters, and invented the Mexican calendar. He returned to the land of the East from which he came, leaving the American coast at Vera Cruz, sailing away into the East (Donnelly). Scott-Elliot, author of the book *Atlantis and the Lost Continent of Lemuria*, agrees that Quetzalcoatl came from the East.
- According to Tracy-Judd, ancient traditions state that the stone edifices near Huamanga were built by a bearded white man, who came there long before the time of the Incas.
- The myths of Poseidon and Quetzalcoatl are practically identical. We find, then, that Poseidon, the culture bringer, arrived some centuries prior to the submergance of Poseidonis (Spence, *The History of Atlantis*).
- Based on many legends, Tracy-Judd believes that Quetzalcoatl, Votan, Itzamua and Kukulcan refer to the same person that entered the Americas from the East.
- The Toltecs of Mexico traced themselves back to Atlan of Aztlan; so did the Aztecs (Bancroft, *Native Races*).

- In a Brazilian legend Samé came across the ocean from the rising sun. Donnelly believes that Zamna of Yucatan may have been the Samé of Brazil. Bochica, the lawgiver of the Muyscas, is said to have had a white beard. He was called the "son of the Sun."
- Donnelly describes a legend of the Indians of the Great Lakes. According to the account, in former times the father of the Indian tribes dwelt toward the rising sun. Having been warned in a dream that a deluge was coming upon the earth, he built a raft, upon which he saved himself and his family and all the animals. He floated upon the waters for several months.
- In the legends of the Iowa Indians and the Sioux Indians, all of the Indian tribes formerly were one and all dwelt together on an island, or at least across a large water toward the east or sunrise (Donnelly).
- There are stories of floods in India, Chaldea, Babylonia, Persia, Greece, Scandinavia, China, among the Jews, Celts, Mexican tribes, North American Indians, and people of Guatamala, Honduras and Peru (Scott-Elliot).
- According to Dr. R. Andree, a German scholar, there are 88 different traditions naming floods. Twenty are of Asiatic origin, five are from Europe, seven from Africa, ten from Australia and the South Sea Islands, and forty-six among the Aborigines of the Americas.

PSYCHIC SOURCES

The Use Of Psychic Channels

Some students may wonder, considering all the negative comments of the Masters concerning the psychic realm, why I would even consider this subject. However, I consider myself not only a student of Ascended Master Teaching, but also a researcher. As such I feel it is my duty to look at every item that may help to bring about a greater understanding of man's history, and in particular, that portion of history that deals with Atlantis.

The Masters minced no words about the psychic realm. They said it contained mankind's destructive, vicious accumulation, and it is the dwelling place of dark forces. It was made very clear to the students how diabolically clever and cunning the dark forces are, how they were successful in misleading students, and in destroying among others, Archangel Zadkiel's Temple near Cuba ages ago. They pointed out repeatedly that it takes an Ascended Being to read the Akashic Records correctly, and that students should not try to make contact with the psychic realm, but should attempt to contact a Master dwelling in the realms of Light. These warnings should be taken seriously.

Yet, I believe there have been and there appear to be now, a few truly gifted psychics who were primarily interested in bringing enlightenment to individuals, and attempted to help mankind as a whole. And this is the yardstick that I propose to be used to measure a psychic. Whenever his work tends to bless mankind, and tends to uplift the race from its bondage, whenever this testimony is given in love and is not aimed at hurting anyone, and that its primary purpose is in helping someone rather than in making money, then I would give this individual a conditional approval, subject to further continuous re-evaluation. In addition I propose to use psychic testimony only to the extent in giving mankind pointers in terms of scientific research, and not in terms of giving instructions on the Law. As far as Cosmic Law is concerned, the Masters have given more than we are able to understand or to apply, yet today.

As one can readily see, my approval of psychics and their spirit guides is rather conditional and selective. In no way do I propose wholesale, indiscriminate contact with the so-called-dead. Except for purposes of scientific research, they should be left alone and not be disturbed.

One of today's psychics would agree to this viewpoint. Aron Abrahamsen, the person employed by J. Goodman during the Flagstaff dig said, "Calling upon discarnates (as a whole other than as individuals) is like opening the floodgates. Some come just to watch. Some are interested in pre-history, some in culture, others had lived in the area." Aron had to learn how to discriminate, and not to pick those spirits who spoke first or the loudest. He had to learn how to tell the difference between the benevolent, the deceitful and the ignorant intelligences. At one time Aron asked for an answer. Many spirits came, prepared to answer. When he stated that only those who really did know need stay — the spirits left one by one. Says Aron, "If you are willing to receive what Uncle Joe (a discarnate relative) has to say, that's what you get. If you are willing to depend on a more universal source, that's what you get!"

The Ascended Masters explained that if an individual transitions from the physical realm, he functions in his memory body, called the soul. He carries over essentially the same type of consciousness he had before. From this explanation we may deduct, if an individual had certain "psychic gifts" and the desire to help mankind before so-called death, then he will carry these attributes forward and he may function as a spirit guide. But as such he has no automatic access to a universal memory bank. He will not all of a sudden become eligible to become a prophet just because he transitioned from the physical world. Cosmic Law does not permit this. Under its rules a person gains access to true knowledge and the universal memory bank only through the old-fashioned way — one must earn it!

Introducing Psychic Sources

Using the yardstick of measurement outlined here-tofore, the first name that comes to mind, is **Edgar Cayce.**

Edgar Cayce is thought by many to have been the greatest clairvoyant in the past 2000 years. He is called the "Sleeping Prophet," because he demonstrated his remarkable psychic gifts while engaged in a self-induced trance. He would simply lie down, fold his arms over his chest and by autosuggestion, go to sleep. While in this state he responded to whatever questions were asked of him. Upon awakening, he remembered nothing of what was said.

Cayce felt that some portions of himself left the physical body during his readings. Was it his etheric body in which he traveled, contacting some memory bank of the past, called the Akashic Records? Cayce said he was contacting the Universal Mind. Occasionally there was some coughing, even when he was in his trance-state. While in this condition he could diagnose the illnesses of people miles away, prescribe treatment for them, or even discuss ancient historical events on Lemuria, Atlantis, and Egypt. During his trance, Cayce could answer the questions of bystanders. Sometimes he spoke in a foreign language, although the only language he knew at the time was English. He could also continue a reading that had been started several years before. He was able to jump quickly from one subject to another, yet he was amazingly consistent in his answers. Cayce did not read books on Atlantis, but gave 350 readings to people who had had a former embodiment on this continent.

Cayce did not give his readings without a great deal of strain. He could give no more than two readings per day, and felt a diet of juices would improve the clarity of his readings. Cayce claimed he had developed his psychic ability over a period of many lives.

In a period of 43 years Cayce gave 14,000 readings, covering 50,000 pages. It was said of him that he was a Bible-reading, God-fearing man. He was not a Saint; he drank occasionally and was a chain-smoker. Cayce transitioned in 1945. All of his readings are preserved by the Association for Research and Enlightenment (ARE) in Virginia Beach.

My own view of Edgar Cayce is this. I believe he was an individual who, through merit earned during former embodiments, was able to partially lift the veil. I deeply respect him for his background and for his attempts to not only give information, but also to spiritually uplift the people to whom he gave a reading. The constant dilemma he faced in trying to figure out a fair charge for his services shows his honesty and sincerity. While his testimony about man's earliest history shows some inconsistency with the information given by the Ascended Masters, his readings of comparable recent events, say beginning 70,000 B.C., is very congruent with that of the Masters. As an example, the Masters spoke of an organized exodus by the initiates just prior to the sinking of Poseidonis. The leaders were given sealed destination orders. Cayce says the same thing, using the phrase, "passports to other countries." By acquainting many individuals with a knowledge of Atlantis and the reality of re-embodiment, Edgar Cayce helped the cause of the Great White Brotherhood immeasurably.

As is the case with many wayshowers, he experienced the wrath of established, orthodox thought. He was arrested twice, once for practicing medicine without a license, and once for fortune-telling. Even so, professional doctors constantly sought his help.

Let us look at other psychic testimony which may be helpful. **Ruth Montgomery**, in her book, *The World Before*, gives us some excellent details about Atlantis, that resemble very much the earlier testimony of Edgar Cayce, and update it to some extent.

Mrs. Montgomery uses as her source, information given by the medium Arthur Ford and ten or twelve other spirit guides, called "Lily and her group." The spirit guides have directed her automatic typewriting for about the last twenty years.

The comments made before about the psychic realm, the correct reading of akashic records, and Edgar Cayce apply very much here. The farther we go back in history, the more difficult it becomes to unfold the leaves of the records. As can be seen in the next section, the testimonies of the psychics under consideration with regard to the early history of man, differ from each other and from that of the Ascended Masters.

As we progress to more recent epochs of history, however, namely to the latter days of Atlantis, the story of the guides match rather well that of the Ascended Masters, and several references are included in the following text. The guides seem genuinely interested in helping mankind, and their message reflects the same urgency as that of the Masters. Both sources agree that time is rapidly running out, and it is up to mankind to reflect upon, and amend, its ways and to turn toward God.

W. Scott-Elliot, through his book *The History of Atlantis and the Lost Lemuria*, makes a valuable contribution, retracing mankind's lost heritage. This book was originally published as two books, one in 1896, and one in 1904. In it Scott-Elliot said that he obtained copies of four more-or-less complete maps of the world during various periods of its history. He claims one map was compiled 75,000 years ago. As his two other sources of information he uses information known to the Theosophical Society, and, in addition, that which he describes as astral clairvoyance.

Concerning this possible source, Scott-Elliot says: "There is no limit to the sources of astral clairvoyance in investigations concerning the past history of the Earth, even with the growth of the planet itself through geological periods which antedated the advent of man. The memory of nature is absolutely accurate and extremely minute." He goes on to say he believes that through training and experience it would be possible for more individuals to do likewise, to become clairvoyant.

The book *Mahatma Letters to A.P. Sinnett* also contains fragments of pre-history. The letters were written by the Masters Kuthumi and El Morya. Based on the way the letters are written, I believe both were unascended at that time. A.D.K. Luk is in agreement they were unascended. This author states that the ascension of the Masters Kuthumi and El Morya occurred in 1888, about six years after the letters were written. Since it has been said by the Masters themselves that only an Ascended Being can read the akashic records accurately, I am placing this book under the category of "psychic sources," as distinguished from information received by Ascended Masters. In addition, this book was written at a time when the occult law was in effect and the Masters were not permitted to convey all of their knowledge. Yet, with all of the limitations that an individual has reading the akashic records correctly, and also considering the effects of the occult law, researchers may do well to study the wisdom contained in this book. With all of its shortcomings, the book contains valuable data, not only with regard to ancient history, but also with regard to the field of natural science.

Psychic Archaeology is a relatively new vehicle as far as investigating our past is concerned. Pioneers of this method are Dr. J. Norman Emerson Ph.D., head of the archaeological department of Toronto University, and Jeffrey Goodman Ph.D., author of the books *Psychic Archaeology* and *American Genesis*.

Psychic Archaeology employs psychics, who in turn tune in to spirit guides. It offers the promise of immediate and spectacular results, and heralds a whole new age of discovery. Dr. Wescott of Drew University, answering critics charging that this new method does not fit into patterns of modern science, asks, "Should scholars deprive themselves of a new way of finding important data, just because they cannot yet explain the methods for obtaining it?"

J. Goodman, in his book *Psychic Archaeology*, explains how psychic archaeology was successfully applied during an exploration at **Flagstaff, Arizona.** Employing the services of the psychic, Aron Abrahamsen, who was assisted by a spirit guide, Goodman was able to find artifacts that many geologists said could not be found in this area. Aron, from his home in Oregon, had selected a ten-foot-square area, telling the scientists where to dig. He even predicted the elevations at which the artifacts were to be found. He was correct in 51 out of 58 specific predictions, giving him an average of 88%. Two distinguished visiting geologists batted a meager 10%. The **Flagstaff** episode challenges the conscience of modern scientists.

Another possible source that may be used in investigating prehistoric events is remote viewing and dowsing. Remote viewing is the ability of a person to describe objects they cannot physically see, through OOBE (out of body experience). The Stanford Research Institute in Menlo Park, California, has done some testing in this area. One person was able through OOBE to locate objects as far away as Lake Victoria, Africa, and the Philippines.

Dr. Alexander Pluzhnikov described how dowsing is extensively used in Russia for archaeological purposes and in discovering minerals. Dowsing is also used by him to locate former underground fortifications, pillars and buildings, both in plan view and elevation. Using motor vehicles, Soviet archaeological dowsers are able to cover an area of ten miles in one hour. When a dowser feels that he has detected a site, further exploration is made on foot. Soviet dowsers also use airplanes to investigate the geology below.

Sheila Ostrander and Lynn Schroeder, who attended a conference in the Soviet Union, and whose book *Psychic Discoveries Behind the Iron Curtain* was a pioneering effort in the field of psychic phenomena, report that the use of dowsing is so wide-spread in Russia, that every combat unit carries a dowser.

In the United States dowsing is not employed as much as it is in Russia, but it is gaining larger acceptance. I was very much surprised when I found out that all of the survey crews of the public agency I work for carry dowsing rods. Several employees of the agency located underground utilities consisting of concrete, clay and steel pipes, two of which were 20 feet deep. Dowsing was also used successfully to locate the end of these underground pipelines.

Jeffrey Goodman advocates a school for second generation research-oriented psychics. Truly gifted people who can give us accurate information about man's origin and history are valuable, indeed.

Early Man On Atlantis

As pointed out in the preceding section, the accounts of the psychics in describing the origin of man differ from each other and from that given by the Ascended Masters earlier in this book.

Cayce describes man, originating as a spirit, not having a physical body. Man as soul, individual consciousness, interrupted an evolutionary pattern by projecting himself into a physical environment. Then, through the use of his creative powers, man became entangled in matter or materiality for selfish purposes to such an extent that he forgot or nearly forgot his divine origin and nature. Based on this account, Edgar Cayce's testimony on the origin of man is by far the closest among all psychic sources, including that which is given in Theosophy, when compared to the account of the Masters, as given through Guy Ballard and Geraldine Innocente.

The spirit guides of Mrs. Montgomery take a different view. They said that mankind originally exhibited "grotesque half human forms." Man's original sin was having sex with animals. As we recall, the Masters said that originally man exhibited total perfection, that this perfection was maintained until the arrival of the laggards, and there were no animals as we know them today.

Scott-Elliot calls the early Lemurian man an animal, destined to reach humanity. "They had not yet received the divine spark which should endow them with mind and individuality."

"It was, we are told, [by whom?] in order that the Manu [guardian of a rootrace] and the Beings [God-like Beings] who aided him might take means for improving the physical type of humanity. The highest type development . . . so far was the huge ape-like creature which had existed on the three physical planets Mars, Earth and Mercury . . . On the arrival of the human life-wave on the Earth, a certain number of these ape-like creatures were found . . . These, of course, joined the incoming human stream as soon as the race became fully physical. Their bodies . . . may have been utilized for purposes of reincarnation for the most backward entities, but it was an improvement of this type which was required and this was most easily achieved by the Manu."

Scott-Elliot, in his description of early man, said that he was of gigantic stature, 12 to 15 feet tall. He had three eyes, one in the back of his head. Where his forehead was there was a roll of flesh; hands and feet were enormous, the heels projected backward. "The figure was draped in a loose robe of skin something like rhinoceros hide, but more scaly, probably the skin of an animal of which we know only of its fossil remains."

Helen Blavatsky, in her book *Secret Doctrine, Vol. II*, adds to this strange tale by quoting as a truth a statement from a book she calls *Secret Book of Dzyan*. She states the second rootrace evolved the SWEAT-BORN, the third rootrace. "The sweat grew, its drops grew and the drops became hard and round. The Sun warmed it, the Moon cooled and shaped it; the wind fed it until its ripeness. The white swan from the Moon overshadowed the big drop." All this in the name of the Masters, who supposedly assisted with the writing of *Secret Doctrine*, the same intelligences who gave teachings through Guy Ballard and G. Innocente. Which message is correct? It is up to the students to decide.

Master Kuthumi, in *Mahatma Letters to A.P. Sinnett*, mentions that the fifth rootrace began its course on the shores of the Central Asian Sea [Gobi-Sea?] one million years ago.

Aron Abrahamsen, the psychic working with J. Goodman, at some time stated that the first inhabitants of America came from Atlantis 500,000 years ago.

Original Limits Of Atlantis

Scott-Elliot described the location of the Atlantean Continent before any destruction occurred. Its northern border started at Labrador; thence easterly to a point south of Greenland, thence continuing easterly to and including Iceland and Scotland; thence southwesterly to a point east of the "Dolphin Ridge;" thence easterly to a point just westerly of the Ivory Coast; thence southwesterly to the westerly line of Brazil; thence northwesterly to Venezuela, Mexico and Louisiana; thence along the westerly line of the Atlantic States of the United States to Labrador. In other words, today's Atlantic States formed the West Coast of Atlantis, and there was land at today's Gulf of Mexico. Scott shows the area west of the Rocky Mountains, and west of a line extending southerly from the Rocky Mountains to a point easterly of the tip of Baja California all part of an island. The westerly border of this island was the present West Coast of the United States and that of Mexico near Baja California.

Edgar Cayce stated that Atlantis, at its prime, consisted of lands between the Gulf of Mexico and the Mediterranean Sea. At that time there also existed lands of today's Nevada, Utah, Arizona, the Gobi Desert and the Sahara Desert. Both deserts were then fertile ground, Cayce said. He designates the Atlantic States of the United States as the West coast of Atlantis, as Scott did.

Ruth Montgomery's spirit guides also gave information on the size of Atlantis. They stated that the Mississippi River formed the West coast of Atlantis, and there was a continuous land bridge eastward towards Portugal and Lybia. The Sahara Desert was then under water and the Nile flowed into the Atlantic. California was the Eastern shore of Mu. In the early days of Atlantis little of Europe was above water.

Atlantean Accomplishments

According to Scott-Elliot, the Rmoahals were the first subrace of the Fifth Rootrace. He describes the government under which the Rmoahals came into existence about 3 million years ago as the most conceivably perfect because it was an Ascended Master who acted as their king. The memory of this divine ruler was preserved, and in later times he was remembered as a God.

Continuing this account, Scott-Elliot next tells of the Tlavatli, who followed the Rmoahals as a subrace. These were taught by adept instructors (highly spiritually-evolved persons), about the existence of a Supreme Being whose symbol was the sun. They developed a sort of sun-worship and built great circles of upright monoliths. These were intended to be symbolical of the sun's yearly course, and were also used for astronomical purposes.

The monoliths were placed so that a person standing at the high altar could observe the rising of the sun during the winter solstice and vernal equinox when standing behind certain stones. In addition, more complex astronomical observations involving more distant constellations were carried out utilizing these stone circles.

In the early days no other image of Deity was permitted other than the sun-disk. It was of gold and was placed in such a way in every temple that it could catch the first rays of the rising sun at the vernal equinox during the summer solstice.

In the great Toltec empire of Mexico, the sun-worship of their forefathers was still the national religion, Scott-Elliot says. The offerings to their beneficient Deity, Quetzalcoatl, consisted of flowers and fruit. It was much later, with the coming of the Aztecs, that the practice of human sacrifices commenced.

All psychic sources went into great detail telling about Atlantean accomplishments in the fields of technology.

Scott-Elliot says that slaves, servants and the lower classes walked or traveled by means of crude carts drawn by animals, but that the more wealthy traveled in airboats which could accommodate eight passengers. The boats were constructed of thin wood or an alloy. They were light in weight and powered in the beginning by personal vril [thoughtforce], with or without mechanical device. In the later days of Atlantis, this manner of propulsion took place by means of an etheric force, operated through mechanical means only. "A strong, heavy, metal chest which lay in the centre of the boat, was the generator. Thence the force flowed through two large flexible tubes as well as through eight subsidiary tubes to either end of the vessel."

The airboat could not travel at great heights. Normally it traveled only a few hundred feet off the ground. It could cross hills, if they were less than

1000 feet high. Seagoing vessels were propelled in a similar manner.

Cayce talks of vehicles that traversed air and water, carrying people to various portions of the land. These vehicles required a navigator. They were lighter than air. The people had the ability to use universal electrical forces for purposes of propulsion of ships and air vehicles.

Ruth Montgomery speaks of a highly-advanced civilization that developed aircraft, submarines, boats and electrical rays similar to today's laser beams. Cayce attributes to the same people the development of radio, TV, transmission of thought through ether, and the reading of and photographing of objects at a distance, even through walls.

Scott-Elliot declares the Atlanteans developed a writing material consisting of thin sheets of metal, having a white porcelain-like surface upon which the words were written. He also states that the Great Pyramid was built 210,000 years ago. It was built to act as a treasure house and shrine in preparation for the submergence of Egypt, which the initiates knew was unavoidable. The cataclysm happened 200,000 years ago. Scott-Elliot also states that Stonehenge was built at least 100,000 years ago, and the Temple at Karnak was built 80,000 years ago.

Cayce speaks of a great civilization in the Gobi Desert, which was more sophisticated than the civilization of Egypt. He gives a much later construction date for the Pyramid, placing it as having been built between 10,490 B.C. and 10,390 B.C.. Cayce says this monument was built by Hermes.

On Atlantis, geologists were able to determine well in advance where an earthquake would occur by applying a formula based on earth pressures and atmospheric pressures (Montgomery).

The Forces of Light and the Forces of Darkness

Scott-Elliot elaborates upon the downfall of Atlantis. He states that the most intellectual and energetic members of the race gradually obtained more insight into the working of nature's laws, and achieved an increasing amount of control over these hidden forces. The use of knowledge for selfish ends, together with lust and brutality, caused terrible catastrophes.

It was a moral question which, from the very earliest of times, divided the Atlantean Race into two hostile camps. The division started in Rmoahal times, three million years ago. It accentuated during the reign of the Toltecs, and it brought the Golden Age under the Toltec Empire to an end, a Golden Age that had reigned for 100,000 years. This came about when, instead of working for the general good of mankind, people allowed selfishness to gain the upper hand.

Scott-Elliot comments on this battle of the forces of Light and darkness, "The battle of Armageddon is fought over and over in every age of the world's history." Not willing to be governed by the wise rule of initiate emperors, the followers of the "black arts" rose in rebellion, and set up a rival emperor who drove the white emperor from his capital, "the City of Golden Gates." However, down to the very end, when Poseidonis disappeared, an Initiate emperor or king — or at least one acknowledging the law of good — had control over some portion of the island continent, acting under the guidance of the Hierarchy, controlling wherever possible, the followers of the dark forces, and instructing the small minority who were still willing to lead pure and wholesome lives.

The adept kings and emperors and the priesthood were all vegetarians!

Edgar Cayce adds much valuable detail. In his readings he calls the followers of the dark forces "Sons of Belial." He said they had no standard they were living up to, except self-aggrandizement. They were desirous of gratifying material emotions and desires. They worshipped ease and pleasure in a material world. During another reading Cayce said the "Sons of Belial" looked upon people as objects or things, rather than highly individualized souls. They were in favor of slave-labor and dealing in gases, liquid air and explosives. They caused the breaking up of land through the use of spiritual truths for material gain, and worked their way into positions of power.

"The Children of the Law of One" were in the other camp. They were complying with the law of love, and were in favor of spreading knowledge of all nature, rather than holding on to the knowledge for themselves to use for personal gain and esteem. The battle between the followers of the two camps started in the very beginning, before the first Atlantean cataclysm, and it continued throughout the history of Atlantis, Cayce said.

Atlantean Wars

The use of explosives was adopted at an early Atlantean period. Scott-Elliot describes grenades that were filled with a most poisonous vapor. Sometimes entire companies of men were destroyed by some bomb which was made to explode over their heads.

At times the air-boats were used for aerial warfare. Up to 100 men could be accommodated. The goal was to upset each other's equilibrium (Scott-Elliot).

Ruth Montgomery speaks of a battle between the Athenians and the Atlanteans, in which the Athenians prevailed. Does this not remind one of Plato?

The Exodus

According to Scott-Elliot, the initiated kings and priests who followed the "good law" were aware beforehand of impending calamities. Each one became a center of prophetic warning, and ultimately a leader of a group of emigrants. In later periods, such as before the Poseidonis cataclysm, the rulers of the country deeply resented these priest-led emigrations, and it became necessary for them to leave secretly during the night.

Cayce speaks of one organized exodus. He states "It had been given out that those that would be saved must journey to the various centers to which the leaders had been given the passports." Migrations took place to Egypt, the Pyrenees, Spain, France, Morocco, British Honduras, Yucatan and Arizona.

Continuing the account of Cayce, he explains that it was through the teachers and the leaders of the Law of One that the people were warned of the coming destruction of Poseidonis. The entity Hept-Supht led in the safe-keeping of the records, which were transferred to the Hall of Records, located near the Sphinx in Egypt. Cayce gives 10,500 B.C. as the date of that activity. The refugees from Poseidonis brought along their superior scientific knowledge. With the cooperation of the rulers of Egypt and the priest Ra-Ta, a period of great advancement in human relations began. There was worldwide dissemination of ideas and knowledge, and there existed institutions for physical and psychic healing. A library of knowledge was set up in Alexandria in 10,300 B.C..

Atlantean Cataclysms

Scott-Elliot states that the destruction of Atlantis took place through a series of catastrophes, varying in character. There were great cataclysms in which entire lands and populations perished, as well as comparatively unimportant landslips such as occur on our coast. These landslips continued to slowly but steadily erode the continent. Four great catastrophes stand out, namely those of 800,000 B.C., 200,000 B.C., 80,000 B.C. and 9564 B.C..

Continuing the account of Scott-Elliot, a portion of the Western and Eastern parts of Atlantis sank during the 800,000 B.C. cataclysm. He calls it a natural convulsion of stupendous character. The Atlantic States became separated from Atlantis. They now formed a part of the United States. The Eastern and Western coastlines of the United States roughly assumed today's shape, except that there was land where the Gulf of Mexico exists today. The west coast of Atlantis was now located about 200 miles east of the Eastern Coast of the United States, and about 1000 miles from the Eastern Coast of Brazil.

The catastrophe which occurred in 200,000 B.C. split Atlantis into two islands. The larger one was called Ruta. Its easterly border included today's Azores. The other island was called Daitya, and was located south of Ruta. Scott-Elliot calls this cataclysm a smaller one.

80,000 years ago there was a large cataclysm, which destroyed all of Atlantis with the exception of Poseidonis, the easterly portion of Ruta. The island was about one-half the size of Australia. According to Scott-Elliot, Poseidonis was destroyed in 9564 B.C..

Cayce talks of three cataclysms. He states that disturbances occurred in 50,000 B.C., then speaks of the "first separation of land," when land portions located at today's Sargossa Sea submerged. It is not clear to me from the reading whether this is connected with the date 50,000 B.C..

The second cataclysm took place in 28,000 B.C., according to Cayce. It separated lands into islands, Poseidia being one of them. Then there was the final destruction, which submerged the "Poseidia Isles," and sank the lands within today's Gulf of Mexico and the Caribbean. Changes along the coasts of Mexico and Central America gave them the shape that exists today.

According to Ruth Montgomery, the first cataclysm occurred in 48,000 B.C.. Volcanoes erupted, and there were tremors "violent enough to fold up the land like a crumpled piece of paper. The world's topography was altered in the twinkling of an eye." The continent of Mu sank to the bottom of the Pacific Ocean. Only Hawaii, Tahiti, Polynesia and a few other islands remained. California attached itself to the Western part of the United States, and the Eastern shoreline of the United States and Brazil assumed today's outline, bordering the Atlantic Ocean. The Bering Strait was formed as a land bridge between Asia and North America.

In North Africa and Europe, the Nile changed course and flowed into the Mediterranean and the Sahara became fertile land. Europe assumed today's shape.

There was a shift in temperature, and tens of thousands of dinosaurs died.

The spirit guides established that the second cataclysm took place in 28,000 B.C.. Lands located in the area of today's Sargossa Sea sank to the bottom of the ocean, and Atlantis split into two islands, called Poseidia and Og. The guides said that the subsidence of portions of Atlantis was initiated by giant underground explosions, the largest ever known on Earth. They also agree with Edgar Cayce that the Biblical flood refers to this cataclysm. Flooding was rampant in Europe as well as parts of the Americas and Africa, but did not affect very much of the Eastern and Southern Hemispheres.

The final cataclysm occurred twelve thousand years ago. Again, it was caused by volcanic action and earthquakes. Only a few islands, such as the Azores and the Bahamas, remained above water. Again there was widespread flooding. "Thus ended the mightiest and most technologically-advanced society ever known to man," commented the spirit guides.

Now let us turn to the *Mahatma Letters to A.P. Sinnett*. In letter No. 23B, the Master Kuthumi wrote Mr. Sinnett in part as follows: "The sinking of Atlantis (the group of continents and isles) began during the Miocene period, and culminated first in the final disappearance of the largest continent, an event coincidental with the elevation of the Alps, and second with that of the last of the fair islands mentioned by Plato. The Egyptian priests of Sais told Solon, that Atlantis, i.e. the only remaining large island, had perished 9,000 years before their time. This was not a fancy date, since they had preserved their records most carefully for milleniums. But then, I say, they spoke but of the 'Poseidonis,' and would not reveal even to the great Greek legislator their secret chronology. As there are geological reasons and a mass of evidence, science has finally accepted the existence of the great continent and archipelago, and thus vindicated the truth of one more 'fable' . . . The deep sea explorations, especially those of the Challenger, have fully confirmed the reports of geology and paleontology. The great event . . . [sinking of Poseidonis] occurred just 11,446 years ago." [This letter was written in 1882. Therefore, according to Master

Kuthumi, Poseidonis sank in 9564 B.C..]

"In the Eocene Age — even in its 'very first part' — the great cycle of the Fourth Race men, the Atlanteans, had already reached their high point, and the great continent, the father of nearly all of the present continents, showed the first symptoms of sinking — a process that occupied it until 11,446 years ago, when its last island, translated into the vernacular as 'Poseidonis,' went down with a crash."

Bibliography, Part II

Barker, A.T. *The Mahatma Letters to A.P. Sinnett.* Wheaton, Illinois, Theosophical Publishing House, 1972

Blavatsky, H. *Secret Doctrine Vol. II* p.206. Wheaton, Illinois, Theosophical Publishing House

Cayce, E.E. *Cayce on Atlantis.* New York, Castle Books, 1968

Churchward, J. *The Second Book of the Cosmic Forces of Mu.* New York, Paperback Library, 1935

vonDäniken, E. *In Search of Ancient Gods.* New York, G.P. Putnam's Sons, 1973

Donnelly, I. *Atlantis the Antediluvian World.* Blauvelt, New York, Rudolf Steiner Publications, 1971

Fell, B. *America B.C.* New York, Pocket Books, 1976

Ferro, R. *Atlantis, the Autobiography of a Search.* New York, Bell Publishing Co., 1970

Goodman, J. *Psychic Archaeology.* New York, G.P. Putnam's Sons, 1977

Goodman, J. *American Genesis.* New York, Berkley Books, 1981

Le Plongeon. *Maya/Atlantis.* Blauvelt, Rudolf Steiner Publications, 1973

Montgomery, R. *The World Before.* New York, Coward, McCann & Geoghegan, 1976

Muck, O. *The Secret of Atlantis.* New York, Times Books, 1978

Nelson, R. *Popul Vuh*

Rehwinkel, A.M. *The Flood.* Saint Louis, Concordia Publishing House, 1951

Scott-Elliot, W. *The Story of Atlantis and the Lost Lemuria.* Wheaton, Illinois 60187, P.O. Box 270, The Theosophical Publishing House, 1972

Spence, L. *The History of Atlantis.* New York, Bell Publishing Co., 1958

Steiger, B. *Atlantis Rising.* New York, Dell Publishing Co., 1973

Tracy-Judd, R.B. *Atlantis, Mother of Empires.* Santa Monica, DeVorss & Co., 1973

Zink, Dr. D. *The Stones of Atlantis.* Englewood Cliffs, 1978

PART III
MAN'S DESTINY

1 - Predictions

SPIRITUAL CHANNELS

The question, "Is it possible to predict the future?" has intrigued the consciousness of man for a long time. Let us begin to answer that question by considering the various factors involved.

The foremost consideration appears to be that on this plane of consciousness, as well as on "the other side" man has free will. Each individual, through his thoughts, feelings and actions sets up causes that influence his future. Generally speaking, then, man is the director of his future activities. This is why it is difficult to project the future. Time also plays a role here, for it is easier to predict what will happen tomorrow, than it is to predict an event ten years hence.

The Master known as Brother Amo, in *Kundgebungen des Eremiten* (Messages of a Hermit) treats the subject of mediumship in great detail. Here are some of his conclusions:

1) Generally speaking, Brother Amo does not advocate magnetizing relatives or other souls by means of seances. The great number of the departed ones should be left alone; they have their own tasks to fulfill. However, there are exceptions. Certain individuals dwelling "on the other side" should be given opportunity to further their own progress and the progress of mankind.

2) Mediums exhibit different levels of purity and consciousness. Genuine mediumship is a gift of God. With this gift comes the responsibility of telling the truth and an obligation not to charge excessive fees. The habits, diet, thoughts, feelings and actions should reflect this responsibility.

3) Not everybody who claims to give a message, gives a correct one. A true messenger needs to be watchful that he does not become the tool of clever dark forces.

4) It takes a great amount of discrimination on the part of the students to recognize higher levels of Cosmic Law and to distinguish between genuine and false messages. The characteristics of a true medium are as follows:

a) The students are not overly praised by the medium through much sweet-talk.

b) There is no condemnation, and there are no threats. Loving suggestions, not orders, are given to the students.

c) There is substance in the message. It is not just empty, repetitive talk.

d) True mediums are humble, simple people, who prefer to stay in the background.

e) They do not charge excessive fees and do not give out certificates of accomplishment.

5) The "second coming of Christ" does not mean that Jesus will reappear and perform a mission similar to His previous one. The "second coming of Christ" is

the repeat of the Christ-message, using true mediums as messengers.

6) Highly evolved Beings, such as Masters, are better equipped than spirit guides to give clear and correct messages. Having achieved mastery on the physical plane, they carry this consciousness "to the other side." A dweller on such a higher plane recognizes patterns and tendencies for the future, set up by certain causes. These patterns, however, are subject to change. They are influenced by the thoughts, feelings and actions of mankind. Therefore, even a Master is not always able to make an accurate prediction of the future, particularly if the future event is far off.

7) Future events can be influenced not only by the thoughts, feelings and actions of individuals and nations, but also by the assistance of an Ascended Master. This assistance must be specifically requested by individuals dwelling on the physical plane, and the request must be accompanied by giving a certain amount of energy to the Master. Masters are also subject to Cosmic Law. In some cases Masters are given to understand that God does not want any interference with the happening of a certain event.

8) In a few years (stated in 1951) it will be possible to have direct contact with the "other side" by means of modern, scientific techniques. This contact will include communication with some departed souls, among them some who will be more evolved. This would make it possible to test the message of a medium. At that time, according to Brother Amo, many mediums will become obsolete. [Such a breakthrough indeed may have occurred. Two-way communications with some of the departed by means of mechanical devices are now possible. Source: MetaScience Research Division, P.O. Box 747, Franklin, N.C. 28734.]

Continuing further on this subject, the Ascended Masters stated that they had to apply for a dispensation to bring the "I AM Activity" into being, and they had to do the same for the "Bridge to Freedom." Only upon being granted these dispensations was it possible for the Masters to bring extensive new information to the students. Also, in both instances there was a period of intense activity, preparing the respective messengers for the task ahead. It was pointed out that both Mr. Ballard and Miss Innocenti had worked with the Masters before, in previous embodiments. This shows that Ascended Masters are also subject to certain rules imposed by higher evolved Beings, and that it is not easy to become an authorized messenger of the Great White Brotherhood.

PREDICTIONS OF THE ASCENDED MASTERS

The Curent Crisis

On rare occasions, Cosmic Law has an overriding effect upon mankind's future. For instance, 2.5 million years ago the Beings responsible for administering the Cosmic Law (as it applies to the Earth) decided to write off the Earth as a worthless experience. As we recall, this was prevented through the kind assistance of Sanat Kumara.

Now we are facing a similar situation. Cosmic Law has decreed that the Earth can no longer delay the first phase of the Inbreath of the Galaxy. We are engaged in a planetary change. All planets of our seven solar systems will move one step horizontally closer to the sun. With the exception of the Earth, there are no other planets with disharmonious conditions within the galaxy. All other planets have long been ready for the Inbreath.

In 1953 Sanat Kumara was informed that within a twenty-year period he had to return to Venus. Within this time-frame the people of the Earth had to increase their collective Light-quota. Failure to do so would mean they would find themselves without a planetary home. The student body of the Bridge to Freedom responded, and through extensive decreeing disaster was avoided. This made it possible for Sanat Kumara to depart for Venus.

Now that the Cosmic Inbreath is at hand, we are again living on borrowed time. We are literally living on a powder keg. In the 1950's the Masters again and again explained this to the students. Their comments follow.

"As the Cosmic Law requires the return of the planets to the suns, and the suns to the Central Sun, each sun begins to regulate its centrifugal force in order to balance the planets belonging to the system."

"As part of the Inbreath, the Earth's axis must be straightened. This must be done gradually and with loving care, so that the large polar ice caps will not be violently displaced. Such displacement would result in the inundation of the continental surface of the planet, which could very well cause the bodily removal of the chelas before the efficacy of their service is manifest."

"The New Age is to enter, even if only one man, one woman, and a five-year-old child are present to greet it."

"We are in the last days. We are in the last great opportunity to set mankind and all life free."

"The Earth has long struggled under the darkness of human hate. It must be cleansed and become self-luminous again." (The substance of the planet was once as luminous as the Sun and is still luminous at its heart-center.)

"Earth is quickening its orbit, and its vibratory action, including that of, the water element and that of the air element, as we prepare for the forward move that will be forthcoming."

"Do you realize what it would mean if the Earth

failed in its expansion of the light as required, in relation to the other planets of this system? You do not know that the intellect cannot comprehend it, but we do. **This is the last effort to free mankind!**"

"The tolerance of the Cosmic Law has reached its limit. It tolerates man's inhumanity to man and man's destructive activity upon man only so long."

"Now we are called upon by the Cosmic Law to make Earth as beautiful as it was in the beginning, TO STRAIGHTEN HER AXIS QUICKLY, and to accelerate the vibratory action of the electrons which make up the atoms of every human being."

"We are engaged in a planetary change, a change that will affect every atom of all so-called matter, even that which seems to be a solid object. That quickening rate of vibratory action in those electrons is constantly going on through and around every individual on the Earth." [From this dictation , which as best I can tell was given in the early 1960's, it appears that the acceleration of the vibratory action of the Earth, including that of its inhabitants, started in the early 1960's. Already in about 1958, the Masters said they had attempted to gradually straighten the axis of the Earth. There was some initial success, but apparently the entire effort was not completed.]

"The long journey of the Earth's evolution is about drawing to its close. The shroud of Earth's pain and agony is being transmuted now into garments of transcendently beautiful light."

"It is the will of God that the Earth's axis shall be straightened and the extremes of climate shall be blended into a habitable balance."

"The Masters are trying to prevent the dangers of cataclysmic activities as the only ways and means of shaking mankind awake. They are attempting to change the axis, melt the ice caps, and raise continents [portions of Atlantis and Lemuria] GRADUALLY AND WITH-

OUT CATACLYSMIC ACTION. From your forcefields is pouring forth a spiritual essence which is acting to transmute the gas belts beneath the earth. These gas belts have caused tremors."

"Mankind has had thousands of centuries to wake up. Life will wait no longer."

"Before mankind today is an assistance as has never been given in the history of the world; because the incoming Golden Age must come in, even if the Earth has to go through a terrific cataclysm."

"For the first time since before the sinking of Poseidonis, this great assistance of Ascended Beings has come forth to the Earth, because the Cosmic Law has said, ′no longer shall we wait for the mankind on Earth. If human beings will not awaken and come into the light and understanding of the Presence now, then nature must do its work.′ You have heard the statement, no doubt, that nature only tolerates mankind′s iniquity so long and then she rises and buries her opponent. That is before you. With sufficient decrees from the octave of the Earth to the Ascended Masters and Cosmic Beings and the mighty I AM Presence, that protection can be given which will MINIMIZE the destructive activity for the Earth. THROUGH THESE CALLS WE CAN DIRECT CURRENTS INTO THE GAS BELTS SO THEY WILL DO THE LEAST DAMAGE." [emphasis added].

Mankind's Last Opportunity

In the previous section we discussed the Divine edict which states that the Earth can no longer delay the progress of the entire galaxy. It was pointed out that we are now engaged in a planetary change, requiring that the inner bodies and the physical vehicles of every individual vibrate above a certain level. Now let us talk about the profound consequences that this Divine edict will have upon mankind.

We have at the present time many members of the fourth rootrace, the fifth rootrace, and some of the sixth rootrace in embodiment. This includes any member of the Angelic Hosts who came out with the fourth rootrace, and of the Guardian Spirits who came forth from other planets at the inception of the fourth rootrace, and any elementals who became "imprisoned" at that time. One Master said, "The Manu of the fourth rootrace is responsible not only for the redemption of all of the members of the fourth rootrace, but also for the redemption of all of the mammals and the animal life, some of which still exist in a state of suspended animation beneath the cap of frozen wasteland (of Siberia)."

All of the members of the sixth rootrace are not yet in embodiment. They can be easily distinguished by the perfection of their forms. They have a perfectly oval face and the majority have golden hair and blue eyes. If they have chosen to serve Lord Himalaya, the Manu of the fourth rootrace, through oriental embodiment, they will take on oriental features. Lord Meru, the Manu of the sixth rootrace, is not yet in embodiment. He will descend when the axis of the Earth is straightened, and the reptiles and insects in South America are redeemed and transmuted. Members of the sixth and seventh rootraces were not allowed embodiment until this time because of over-population, caused by re-embodiments of the same lifestreams.

At this critical juncture, all of mankind's ten billion lifestreams will be given a last chance to make amends, and to give manifest expression to man's destiny as a co-creator with God. According to the Masters, a plan has been accepted that provides a last opportunity for all of mankind. Under this plan, those that are presently in embodiment will have their last opportunity to turn to God. Those who are not embodied will be allowed one final embodiment. The Masters said the following about this event, "The cycle where an individual is reassigned in the Halls of Karma, given new opportunity to serve and, at the proper moment to pass through the gates of birth, has closed."

According to the account of the Masters, there will be a division of mankind, and only those who make a conscious effort to improve their habits, their thoughts, feelings and actions will be allowed to return to Earth for a new embodiment. Before we deal with the question of what happens to those, who by reason of their conduct forfeit the right to use the Earth as their planetary home, let us pause briefly and reflect upon the criteria that will be used to make this decision.

It should be clear from the outset, that man will not be judged upon the basis of religious affiliation, race or color. Also, knowing the law without applying it, is insufficient. Pure motives, a correct attitude, and willingness to put into practice what one knows, alone are omnipotent. Our conduct in meeting the problems of everyday life, in constructively qualifying energy, and contributing to the good of all, opens the door.

Now let us talk about those, who by their own choice, refuse to make the necessary adjustments.

Throughout the years 1959 to 1961 the Masters announced the creation of two new planets, one of which was named Excelsior. [Some dictations use the word "foci, or orb." Therefore, this place of abode may not fit the ordinary definition and the characteristics of a planet.] The purpose of one of the planets was to serve as a future home for those in this embodiment who continue to refuse to make the necessary effort to improve themselves and turn to God. The other planet was to be used by elementals. Here are the messages as they were given at that time by the Masters.

"Why should the Earth, so long a schoolroom not only for her own evolutions, but for the laggards from the other stars as well, be cluttered up by the same lifestreams who have been given opportunity through aeons of time to learn the same exact lesson, when there has been already created for them a beautiful new planetary schoolroom, where they can take their own sweet time in learning this lesson. This new schoolroom (star) is as shining and beautiful as the Earth herself was when it was designed by Helios and Vesta for approximately 3 1/2 billion lifestreams.

"We are entering a new cycle now, wherein the seventh rootrace shall quickly have expression on Earth, wherein every laggard that is in embodiment on Earth shall, at the close of this embodiment, never take embodiment here again; wherein every lifestream, particularly those who are dedicated by mouth but not by heart to the cause of Light, who will not accelerate the vibratory action of his inner and physical vehicles, at the close of this embodiment, shall not again enter upon this Earth star. To this end we have arranged a separate little star, where they can accelerate themselves at leisure and take as long as they like."

"Those who do not choose to accelerate the vibratory action of their energy shall find hospitality on another star, but the planet Earth and the few who are willing shall go forward to freedom."

"We are creating another planet where you shall have great opportunity to serve. As yet, We have not directed the Cosmic Ray through it, to set in into motion. It is a planet to be inhabited particularly by elemental life which has not yet achieved its full freedom on this Earth.

"There are a lot of lovely beings on Excelsior; there is also that other planet created for those of you who wish to sleep on or [are content to] move with the vibratory action of the present Earth people. BUT BY GOD, those who remain on this Earth are going to vibrate like those beings who represent the seventh rootrace, and this Earth shall return to the beauty and perfection it had in the beginning. The laggards can go. Incidentally, some of the original laggards the Earth took on a long time ago are now more spiritually advanced than some of the Earth's original guardian spirits."

" . . . having stood sponsor for you before the Karmic Board, having had to create Excelsior and living thereon for no little time — a lovely planet, but cramped a bit, I might say, and I (El Morya) shall be glad when the student body takes over their opportunity to bring in the Golden Age here on Earth and I can go to Mercury and remain. Excelsior is a shiny little planet and its inhabitants are lovely and I enjoyed making it . . ."

Note: Volume 1, No. 3 "Law of Life Enlightener" issued by A.D.K. Luk Publications tells of a separate place, focus or planet called Polaroid, where some of the Earth's present laggards will be given more time to accelerate their vibrations.

Nations of Destiny

America, the Grail of Light

The Masters stated repeatedly that North America is to be the heart center of the "Permanent Golden Age" that is now dimly touching the horizon. It was in North America that the first lifestreams embodied upon the planet Earth. At the completion of his journey, mankind again will connect with the place from which he started.

"America's destiny was seen and planned from the beginning. We look upon the United States as the

Ascended Master Nation of the Earth, whose Threefold Flame becomes the magnet to raise every other nation into the eternal perfection of the octave of the Ascended Masters.

"Here is the only spot on Earth where there is a chance of establishing this great perfection, for America has not been drenched in human blood. Europe has been saturated with human blood for countless ages, (including the ages when it was part of Atlantis). All great wars upon this planet took place on both sides of North America. Great war devastations also took place on Lemuria.

"Once when a great civilization had reached its apex in America, it used the flag you are using now."

"The vast plains east of the Rocky Mountains will one day be teeming with semi-tropical vegetation, and its people will live in peace and abundance."

"This country has a tremendous concentration of vital energy within it, by reason of the fact that here was the initial pulsation in the world of form. This very vital force has enabled it to come so far in so few centuries.

"In your beloved America, in the not-so-far-distant future will come forth a recognition of the Real Inner Self (the I AM Presence) and her people will express high attainment. She is a land of light and her light shall blaze forth, brilliant as the sun at noon day, among the nations of the Earth. She was a land of great light ages ago, and will come again into her spiritual heritage, for nothing can prevent it.

"A perfect form of government will come, when you have cast off certain fetters within, that hang like fungi and sap your strength. Beloved ones in America, be not discouraged, when the seeming dark clouds hang low. America shall fulfill her destiny, another Golden Age shall reign upon earth, and it shall be maintained for an aeon.

"The plan for the Permanent Golden Age is already

finished at inner levels; many of you, we trust, will be the builders. That definite design shall be fulfilled regardless of all of the appearances of this hour [this dictation was given just before W.W. II.] There is no such thing as escaping its fulfillment. It could come so much sooner if the people would awaken and would send us more calls for this Light."

Other Nations of Destiny

In addition to those in America, the peoples of Egypt, China, South America and Germany were singled out by the Masters to make a valuable contribution to the Permanent Golden Age.

"Out of Egypt came forth, in an earlier cycle, very great Light, and out of Egypt will again come — Very Great Light."

"China has yet a great service to fulfill for the planet Earth."

In *Explanations of the Hermit* and *Messages from the Hermit*, a Master reminds Germans, and those of German descent, of the holy task they are to perform. They are to be the heralds and missionaries of the divine plan for the Earth. "Because of the characteristics of the German mind, which exhibits a persistent, never-ending quest to seriously and sincerely look for causes and solution, Germans, like no other people in the world, are capable of understanding the nature of God."

South America will receive increased importance because it is here that the seventh rootrace shall find embodiment. The first members of the seventh rootrace were selected in June of 1954, and the Masters stated that the entire first subrace was ready to embody in October 1960. Now we are entering a cycle wherein the seventh rootrace shall quickly have expression on Earth.

"When the seventh rootrace enters, all members will be found to be equipped with magnificent voices, all will be able to both precipitate and levitate at the time of birth, and they will have the knowledge of the heavenly realm.

"The seventh rootrace is due to come forth for the most part in South America; some will arrive in North America. We have chosen South America because across Brazil and throughout that country, which is now jungle, the earth has had some time to rest."

"Within the very Earth itself, down to about fifteen feet below its surface, from Peru to the Amazon, along the Amazon to Rio de Janeiro, an activity of the Violet Flame has been established. This will result in a great number of poisonous reptiles being spewed forth into the Amazon and then out into the ocean. The color of the Amazon will turn to a beautiful sapphire blue. Some of the members of the first subrace of the seventh rootrace went before Mother Mary in May 1961 . . . and I am quite sure that 1000 or 2000 will take embodiment primarily on the North American continent, because as yet the South American Continent is not ready. When mature, the members of the seventh rootrace will look distinct from all others. Their hair will be amber, they will have a seraphic face, slender figures, long limbs and long tapered fingers. The women will look like Goddesses. The seventh rootrace consists of one root and has seven branches, only they do not flower all at once."

The Rising of Atlantis

The Masters stated that portions of Atlantis will rise, and when they do, they will appear in their original beauty.

"There will be seen hermetically sealed temples made of a crystalline substance. Two or three cities that belonged to Atlantis during her prime are being very gradually raised right now from the ocean floor. We are hopeful that this will occur in an equally unobtrusive manner as the axis change continues (September 1957).

"It was hoped that the axis could be straightened out by September 15, 1958." [This goal was not accomplished.]

Future Discovery of Records

The Ascended Masters gave various references with regard to the future findings of records. Because of the importance of these references, some are given verbatim.

"The cosmic record that has been written in every civilization has been transferred, preceding the usual cataclysmic action into this cosmic library. They are kept in their original form within the electronic belt around the Central Sun."

"We have always the etheric record, which is the counter part of the outer record. The etheric record is absolutely accurate. From it we make reliable records on sheets of gold. This activity has been going on for thousands of years. We took all important records from the Alexandria Library before it was burned. We also have the important records of the Vatican."

"The physical records of each civilization, written in the language of that civilization, are stored at the Royal Teton Retreat."

"In one Retreat a complete record of any civilization that was on Earth is kept. The entire record is on scrolls.

"The records in the Teton Retreat are stored within metal containers and are attached to spindles of a ten-inch length. The records are etched by something like a stylus on eight-inch-wide ribbons of pressed gold, no thicker than ordinary writing paper. The gold contains some other alloy to make it tough and pliable. The length of the ribbons is from seven to fifty feet. The characters of the records appear similar to script.

"There were many Krishnas who came to Earth. The first Krishna left written documents which survived many catastrophes, and which had to be moved across the face of the Earth. Several of the original documents are kept at Himalayan monasteries. The records were made by coating rolls of linen with a soft wax and then inscribing Krishna's message. The wax was allowed to harden, yet it was still pliable. Finally, the roll was placed on two spindles. Some scrolls are several hundred feet long."

"Priceless scrolls and scripts on parchment and stone have been transported from Tibet to the Andes. Future civilizations will enjoy these magnificent treasures.

"Records of Atlantis are now resting on the bed of the Atlantean Ocean. They are in a state of perfect preservation, and will be brought forth in the future by Ascended Beings who directed their preparation and protection.

"The focus at Darjeeling was established 1000 years ago. Because of El Morya's interest in interstellar space, an observatory was established to study stars and planets. Here are priceless charts which one day will be released for the illumination of mankind."

"The library at the Ascension Temple at Luxor contains priceless books from every civilization. Many of the books that people thought were burned at Alexandria during that fire at the library as well as parchments from early ages are kept here."

"The Blue Lotus Retreat in the Himalayas contains the writings of all ancient sages. They will be released when there is no more selfishness, and when people will value this spiritual wealth."

"The records going back to Mu are preserved and shall come forth again for the benefit of the seventh rootrace, when South America is purified of all effluvia of past mistakes, when the Earth is straightened on its axis, and when the jungles and morasses of Brazil and the Amazon River are purified and made habitable."

"In one cave in India the most ancient records upon this Earth are still held in safe-keeping. Because of lack of spiritual growth and understanding by mankind these records will not be brought forth at the present time."

"The Ascended Masters always foresaw destructive cataclysms and preserved all important records. One day, when humanity is prepared for it and when it is positively safe for these records to be given to the outer world, there will appear in a central location a marvelous library, not made by hand, where these records will be available, and those in the outer world who have received the necessary credentials, may see them."

Other Predictions of the Masters

The following quotations on miscellaneous subjects are based on dictations by the Masters of Wisdom.

"Another avatar was due long since, but was not able to come because of the slow development of the human race."

"The people of the Earth in this present hour are looking again for a second coming of Christ, which is imminent, and I have already prepared the new

Christus, who but awaits the proper benevolent moment for this event." (Lord Krishna, 1961)

"Women will assume an increasingly important role in the future. They will be restored to the dignity which they experienced in the early Golden Ages. Now as the Earth is entering the Permanent Golden Age the Feminine Ray in the Andes will become predominant. Gradually it will be more and more noticeable that the spiritual aspirants will turn their attention to the Andes Mountains rather than to the Himalayas."

"As humanity becomes more harmonious and pure, all animals will disappear from the Earth. Even weeds will be no more and the Earth once again will return to her pristine purity described as the Garden of Eden."

"All racial characteristics will eventually fade out, and all will blend into the Aryan type, in features and color. Color is only in the physical body. The Christ-self of all is blazing white."

"On Atlantis the flames kept in the temples represented the virtues of God. People visited the temples to regain their strength. That day shall come again in the not-too-distant future. During Atlantean times, at the end of an embodiment, the body was placed in the flame and it disappeared instantly. This will come again."

"New inventions are ready to be given to mankind. These include airships which will receive energy for propulsion from the atmosphere. They also include geologists' equipment and astronomical equipment."

"Great Master Chemists have been working for the past fifty years. After America's final crisis, her people will be taught the use of universal energy for light, heat and power. This will come forth in still greater perfection than has ever been known in any previous age." (Written in about 1932.)

"It is our cause to redeem the Earth quickly, restore it to perfection and bring mankind again into conscious communication with the Angelic Host and the transmuted happy Elemental Kingdom, bringing in the Golden Age. It shall be a permanent and shining star indeed. 'Freedom's Holy Star,' it shall be called, and again the love and light that flows to it and through it will make it one of the brightest of the stars in this system."

"The sinister force attempting to create chaos and destruction will be completely destroyed. When that is accomplished, the mass of humanity will turn to the Great God Presence. Peace will reign on Earth, and man will send out good will to man."

The Masters admonished the students not to rest their attention upon the Biblical story of Armageddon. They stressed that this great tragedy is avoidable. The attention and active visualization given to a prediction of a destructive event uses energy that may better be used for constructive purposes. It also enhances the chances of a probability of the occurrence of such an event.

This warning may apply also to other forecasts of a destructive nature. The dire predictions by psychics cited in the next sections are primarily shown to serve as a warning. These catastrophes, or most of them, do not have to happen. They could happen if mankind persists in the pursuit of so-called happiness. These events may still be averted or at least the loss of human life and the chaos may be held to a minimum. As discussed earlier, the most effective way of averting them is through the forming of decree groups.

PREDICTIONS OF THE PSYCHICS

Edgar Cayce predicted that indications of lost civilizations would be found in the Atlantic Ocean, in the

Gobi Desert, in the hills of Iran, and in the jungles of Indonesia. He also stated that certain Atlantean records were preserved at locations off the coast of Florida, in Egypt, in a hall of records located near the Sphinx, and in Yucatan. According to Cayce, these records would be found during future earth changes or during the period previous to them. They not only contain early Atlantean records, but also the history of the building of the Great Pyramid.

Ruth Montgomery's spirit guides (*The World Before*, written in 1976) agree with the location of Atlantean records near the Sphinx. They stated that these records are located so deep within the earth that it would take some forty-eight workers an entire year to reach them.

These guides predict that China will fulfill an important role in the future. They foresee that it will become more democratic than Russia, and that it eventually will become a world leader.

Exciting things will happen in the field of alternate energy. Ruth Montgomery's spirit guides foresee that new forms of energy will be produced by solar disks that slowly rotate in wide arcs while generating steam for power. These will be located near large industrial areas and transformers will be propelling machines and harnessing energy. This new form of energy will also be available for cars. A way of storing solar energy, as in ancient Atlantis, will revolutionize the power industry.

Edgar Cayce states that great earth changes are to take place within the time period of 1958 to 1998. He forecasts that the United States will be one of the areas of the globe to experience such physical changes. He speaks of a breaking up of the earth in the western region, disturbances in the central portion, and even greater changes on the North Atlantic Seaboard and on the southeastern coastline. The disturbances on the West Coast and on the southeastern coastline will happen sooner than those that will affect the area around New York City. Waters of the Great Lakes will empty into the Gulf of Mexico. All these changes, Cayce maintains, will take place on a gradual basis as part of the earth changes in North America. Areas that will not be affected will be Ohio, Indiana and Illinois. Land will appear off the east coast of America, in the Pacific and in the Caribbean Sea.

Turning to Canada, Cayce predicts that Western Canada will be disturbed, but that much of southern and eastern Canada will remain safe areas. South America will be shaken from its northernmost portion to its southern tip.

According to Cayce, these earth changes will be preceded by disturbances in the South Pacific or in the Mediterranean and Aetna area. Ruth Montgomery's spirit guides predict that the San Andreas fault, which parallels the California Coast, will split in a few years, and that the portion of California closest to the Pacific will sink into the ocean. Some of California will survive, the guides say. Rumblings below the earth should be considered as warnings. Before this event, which is to take place "in the next few years," Vesuvius will erupt with great gushings of lava.

The guides call the shift of the Earth's axis unavoidable. This shift is supposed to occur at the close of this century. At the time of the shift of the axis, Manhattan Island, and other sections of the East Coast as far north as Newfoundland, will vanish. Florida, as well as other areas of the globe, will also be gravely affected. On the embers of a devastated civilization will arise a better one, a civilization which will emphasize the brotherhood of man. This will be followed by one thousand years of peace.

2 - Leadership

INTRODUCTION

The Masters made it very clear that the time for the first phase of the Inbreath is at hand. Cosmic Law will wait no longer. We are facing certain planetary changes that will affect each of us. A new time period, a time period which can no longer be postponed, is ahead of us. This period will begin, regardless of whether of not it must be entered with only one woman and one man. We are facing a planetary crisis which can either be accompanied by catastrophic natural disasters, or it may occur in a less violent manner. Which do we prefer? This question is a question which must be answered NOW.

Having discussed the plan of the Masters Saint Germain and El Morya, and their blueprint for a better tomorrow, the next question would be, "Who is best qualified to lead the human race out of its present bondage? Who should direct the effort to create **One**

Nation under God, the group activities and the research centers the Masters talked about? should the leaders of today be the leaders of tomorrow?"

These are not easy questions to answer. Time and time again well-meaning individuals have attempted to bring enlightenment to mankind, only to be frustrated by the limited consciousness, lack of humility, and personal ambition of those who did not see the vision, and who thereby curtailed the original effort.

In an attempt to answer the questions at hand, let us turn to dictations of the Ascended Masters, as they pertain to the leaders of today in the fields of religion and science.

CHRISTIAN CHURCHES

As can be seen from the following quotations, the Masters were extremely critical of the conduct of today's orthodox Christian Churches.

"The churches have had the opportunity for two thousand years to set mankind free. Yet the people have grown into greater and greater bondage. When the light of God comes forth through two humble human beings [Mr. and Mrs. Ballard], that which is supposed to represent the Christ turns its destructive forces upon them." (Goddess of Liberty, June 1938)

"Observe my experience in leaving the example of the Ascension to mankind, how little good it did. Three hundred years afterwards the Great Truth was so obscure that mankind scarcely understood anything of the achievement or the example which I left. Instead, there was concentration on the crucifixion; there was always that vicious force in the world which wanted to destroy the Light." (Jesus, November 1939)

"Because of the many translations, the *Bible* is hardly recognizable compared to what its reality was in the beginning. Everything suffers through translation, for human opinions are always imposed upon the original." (Bob Singleton, March 1938)

Many modern researchers are of the opinion that several key elements of the *Bible*, such as references pertaining to karma and reembodiment were changed or omitted during several conventions of the early Christian church.

During Cortez´ conquest of Mexico, many bishops destroyed every scrap of writing they could find. Bishop Landa´s stay in Yucatan and his fanatical destruction of all Mayan records caused an irretrievable loss to man´s intellectual advancement and to mankind´s progress in general.

Churches advise, "Just believe in Jesus Christ and you will be saved." When people reach "the other side" they will find this is not so. Is a mere belief in a Master sufficient to transmute the causes set up by mankind´s wrong thoughts and actions?

Which church leaders have looked beyond the *Bible* to look for life after life or which one dared to do explorations to look for the origin of man, or try to investigate the claims for ancient continents such as Atlantis of Lemuria?

Clearly, our established Christian Churches, as well as some other religious groups, have failed us in providing enlightened leadership during the past ages. They were given opportunity after opportunity; they have been found wanting.

MODERN SCIENCE

Next let us take a look as to what type of leadership we might expect if we follow the leaders of modern science, including our conventional historians.

According to our historians, and what is taught to

our youngsters in school, about 7000 years ago, some nomads and hunters gave up their clubs and moved from their caves and tents. Primitive tribesman suddenly becamc skilled and created a miraculous city state in the Mesopotanian Valley. They constructed astronomical observatories, charted the stars accurately, built pyramids, temples and modern homes, became skilled in cuneiform (wedge-type) writing and produced experts in the field of ceramics. One must ask, where did the cavemen, hunters and food-gatherers obtain this sudden knowledge?

Continuing the account of our experts, the Neanderthal man disappeared suddenly 40,000 years ago and modern man (Cro-Magnon) appeared, without a period of transition. The generally-accepted theory of evolution falls silent at its crucial moment, the birth of modern man. Darwin's theory remains an unproven hypothesis because the "missing link" is still missing.

Professor J. Goodman states that the only reason archaeologists investigated Atlantis was to disprove the belief that there ever was such a continent. Does this sound like a search for enlightenment, new knowledge and truth?

Another example of the type of help we may expect from some modern scientists was recently experienced at Bimini. When a geologist was asked to comment on the rectangular stone patterns on the ocean floor he responded, without hesitation, that they were caused by wave action. Of course, one knows the waves of the Atlantic Ocean are very sophisticated. They even cut out neat rectangular joints in the stones. According to our friends, the modern scientists, plowshares in New England have similar abilities. Ancient letters carved in stone and photographed in the book *America B.C.* by Barry Fell, a professor at Harvard, are explained away as markings of plowshares.

Commenting on the efforts of modern scientists, Mark Twain states, "There is something fascinating about science. One gets such wholesome returns from a trifling investigation of facts."

Sir Fred Hoyle, an eminent British scientist, has mounted a new assault on the Darwinian evolutionary theory, saying the possibility of its being true is "so utterly minuscule" as to be absurd. He arrives at a probability of one to 10 to the 40,000th power, or one followed by 40,000 zeros. In effect, he says, the chances are nil, so "outrageously small" it would be incredible "even if the whole universe consisted of organic soup."

Modern developments in microbiology have "made it overwhelmingly clear that the truth is quite otherwise," says Sir Fred Hoyle in his book, *Evolution from Space*, published by Simon and Schuster. Hoyle, knighted by Britain for his scientific contributions, has headed the Royal Astronomical Society. Hoyle adds, "Every competent space mathematician would assure you that such a Darwinian idea had no chance of working . . . Every computer expert will, in fact, assure you that throwing random mistakes into a computer is no way to improve it."

We had enough money to go to the moon. This program cost the United States ten billion dollars. Why can't the government invest ten million dollars to research the origin of man?

Let us take a look at the field of geology. Geology may be defined as a study of the structure, the history and the development of the Earth and its inhabitants as revealed by rocks. The basic claim is made that fossils may be found up to a depth of 50,000 feet, and the oldest rocks are found at the bottom. However, according to geologist Professor Rehwinkel, there is no place on earth where sedimentiary rocks of such thickness can be found. We never have to go down more than a few thousand feet before we strike the bedrock of granite, and below this no fossils are found.

Rehwinkel backs his contention with a picture of nine actual drilling samples taken at different locations in the United States. They show that in seven cases the rocks that, according to the geological column, were the oldest, were actually found on top, forming sort of an upside down cake. Rehwinkel concludes, "Geology is anything but a science!"

T.C. Chamberlin, called the dean of American geologists, admits that it is not possible to proceed directly through the whole succession of bedded rocks, but that different layers of the different ages may be encountered due to workings, tiltings or wearing away. The full series of strata is discovered only by combining the data which is to be found at several locations. Even if this is done, an absolutely complete series cannot be put together. In other words, this ingenious geological timetable, consisting of the various series of rocks and species with the oldest rocks and fossils to be found on the bottom, is purely a theory and hardly exists anywhere.

Dr. Price, the author of many books on geology, concludes that the theory of evolutionary geology cannot be considered as science, but is a mere theory, a hypothesis, a belief. Its claims cannot be verified as scientific proof.

ANCIENT ACCOMPLISHMENTS

When one is determined to search, it becomes readily apparent that the wisdom and technology of the past surpassed the accomplishments of our present time in many fields.

Livio Stechini, a professor of ancient history, describes some of the features of the Great Pyramid of Giza, one of the Seven Wonders of the World.

1) It serves as a calendar by which the length of

the year can be measured to the exact minute.

2) It incorporates the value of Pi (the constant by which the diameter of a circle must be multiplied to calculate its circumference).

3) It is so precisely aligned with the North Pole that modern compasses can be adjusted to it.

4) The measurements of its sides and angles incorporate the circumference and radius of the Earth — even accounting for polar flattening.

5) Some of the stones of the pyramid, weighing many tons, are fitted together so perfectly that the joints are no wider than the thickness of silver paper.

There are other accomplishments attributed to Ancient Egypt. The Nile was diverted to build the city of Memphis. The artificial lake of Moeris was created as a reservoir of the Nile. It is 450 miles in circumference and 350 feet deep.

Commencing in 1953, S. Mercer, Professor Emeritus of Egyptian languages at the University of Toronto, spent six years completing translations of the hieroglyphs carved into five small pyramids near Sakkara, Egypt. The hieroglyphs, considered to be the oldest written records of mankind, reveal that Egyptian children were already taught in 2100 B.C. that the Earth was round. Their curriculum included astronomy, medicine, and engineering.

According to Donnelly, these Egyptians possessed gold and silver money. They manufactured a linen so fine in quality in 600 B.C., that a single thread of garment had 365 minor threads. The word "chemistry" comes from chemi, and chemi means Egypt. Their dentists filled teeth with gold. The "papyrus of Berlin" is at least 6,700 years old. There is no indication of an early period of savagery or barbarism. The carpenters´ and masons´ tools of today are almost identical with those used in ancient Egypt.

In 1900 a Greek sponge diver took an object from the wreckage of an ancient vessel. Fifty-eight years later, Dr. Price, of the Institute of Advanced Studies at Princeton, discovered the object to be a 2000-year-old instrument, namely, a sextant to measure the solar system. A series of calibrations and inscriptions explained the theory of the instrument.

How does modern science explain the mysterious geometric patterns on the ground surface near Nazca, Peru? Many believe they are ancient landing strips. The Peruvians built roads 2000 miles in length. They built aqueducts up to 500 miles long. Suspension bridges were built by them thousands of years before they were introduced in Europe. A structure was built at Cuelap, in Northern Peru, that originally was 3600 feet long and 300 feet high. The Inca fortress of Sacsayhuaman contains a monolithic granite block thirty-nine feet high, polished and ground, weighing more than 100 tons.

At Baalbeck, Lebanon, stone blocks were found to be sixty feet long, weighing up to 2000 tons. No crane of today is able to lift such a weight. The stones were beautifully shaped, and had perfectly square corners.

After fifty years of research, the German archaeologist, A. Posnansky, concluded that the city of Tiahuanaco was at least 10,000 years old.

According to Dr. Mae Neish, archaeologist for the Peabody Foundation, the Teohuacan Valley, about 100 miles south of Mexico City, was first occupied in about 10,500 B.C.. When I visited this place in 1972, I noticed that the interior remains of some buildings still contained some beautiful wall paintings that had been done in vivid colors. These had hardly faded over a period of several thousand years. Also, the stone-sculptured feathered serpents still showed remarkable detail and good proportion.

How does modern science explain the 200, sixty-feet-high stone figures on Easter Island, weighing fifty tons each, or the Mayan observatory built at Chichen

Itza in Yucatan? Does it have an explanation for the Piri Reis map of the world of 1513, called incredibly accurate by a cartographer of the U.S. Navy? It shows coastlines and islands of the Antarctic that were not discovered until 1953. Charles Hapgod, a cartographer, concluded that this map was based on the modern Mercator projection, and it required the knowledge of spherical trigonometry.

Archaeologists did find small, highly-polished magnetic mirrors at one of the oldest sites in Mexico. These mirrors were ground to the precision of optical lenses. No one knows what they were used for.

Near North Salem, in the Northeastern part of the United States, a ninety-ton capstone was found to be supported by five vertically placed pegstones.

Does all this sound like the work of cavemen, food-gatherers, hunters, shepherds and savage warriors, as most of our modern scientists claim?

Why is the theory of evolution, or any other hypothesis, being taught in public institutions and shown over public television, without mentioning the possibility of man's creation by a highly-evolved, intelligent Being? We cannot agree with an existing pattern that accepts new evidence only if it falls in line with a certain pre-assumed path, with hardly anyone asking questions, hardly anyone critically examining the other's evidence, and where all are happy because they found a new "fact" contradicting creation by a Superior Being.

It takes brave men to breach the status quo and endure the ridicule of one's colleagues, but a new beginning must be made. We do not condemn modern science for not having the answers to many of mankind's concerns, but we must question why established modern science has no serious intent in seeking answers, and why it insists upon ridiculing the effort of those who are reporting other theories without bias.

Therefore, since both the orthodox churches and modern science are unable at this time to provide effective leadership, we must look elsewhere!

THE LEADERS OF TOMORROW

The Masters stated that students of Ascended Master teaching are best qualified to be the leaders in the Golden Age. "They are the ones who know best about Life and the Laws of Life and how to deal with the difficult situation the Earth is now faced with." These students know best how to deal with the opposition — the forces of darkness. They know how to protect themselves from negative influences, and how to invoke the assistance of the Great ones through the powers of magnetization, precipitation, visualization and the spoken word.

They are best equipped to restore the sacred relationship of religion and science, which were thought of as ONE during ancient times. They know best how to face the tomorrow. The students, in turn, need to be receptive and tune into the loving counsel and guidance of the Ascended Masters. These are the real leaders, They know the best way to bring in the Golden Age, and They know best how to face the obstacles that lie ahead. Without the assistance of the Ascended Masters there would be no hope for the world. With the assistance of the Ascended Masters and the sincere, determined effort of a few students, victory is assured.

In discussing the requirement of the pioneers of the future, the Masters indicated they do not expect perfection overnight. "When a baby attempts to walk and it falls down," they said, "it tries again." This is the type of action the Masters expect from the chelas, that of TRYING to work to the best of their ability.

However, it was made clear that those who wish to set an example should be free from habit-forming drugs, alcoholic drinks, and smoking. They encouraged the students to look at the advantages of a vegetarian diet.

In this New Endeavor there is no such thing as passive membership; all members must assume an active role. Students should help wherever they can. In this teaching there are no leaders and no followers, all are an important member of a team. That team must pull in one direction towards a common goal.

Different aspects of truth, designed to meet the requirements of the hour, have been presented for centuries by members of the Great White Brotherhood. Saint Germain's dispensation of the 1930's and El Morya's and Saint Germain's dispensation of the 1950's were designed to meet today's conditions, and they represent the latest of these activities. The teachings of these most recent efforts stand on their own, needing no other teaching or religion for reference or verification. The Masters emphasized that the information They gave during that period is at least ten times that which is needed for mankind's ascension.

Students of these instructions cannot mix or blend the original dictations of the Masters with other teachings, and expect to get harmonious results. Mixing different presentations of Truth only creates confusion. One cannot pick and choose what one likes about the instructions of the 1930's and 1950's and blend them together with other teachings, just as one cannot graduate from a university if one chooses to take courses that do not meet the requirements for a degree. Likewise, students need to make a decision and elect to stay with one particular group.

The common bond of love and respect for the Ascended Masters and co-workers will help to overcome the difficulties that lie ahead. Much will be required from a few; it always has been that way. Group leaders and members need to daily protect themselves from negative influences. This is done by either decreeing or contemplation and communion with the I AM Presence. Jesus said in July, 1954: "My ministry was one of action. Every day before I left the house, great numbers of people had gathered — primarily to receive relief from all manner of discomfort and disease of mind and body. Very few came to learn the application by which I had achieved such powers to give surcease from distress. I had learned **never**, under any circumstances, to go forth to serve until I had first ANCHORED my consciousness, feeling and self in the PRESENCE OF GOD. Only when I was firmly established in that unshakable faith, that indestructible fortress of His Power and Presence, would I endeavor to convey that consciousness of His Goodness, through words and works, to my fellowman. Earnest men and women, filled with zeal and enthusiasm, often rush forth without such personal contemplation and communion with the Godself."

By serving, helping others and by passing the various trials in everyday life one gains the merit that is needed to be initiated for the higher tasks ahead. There are no diplomas, no titles and certificates of accomplishment. The Ascended Master Mary urged the students, "be humble in your knowledge."

Right motives and the determination to serve God and the Ascended Masters to the best of one's understanding, keeping the original message of the Masters pure and unchanged, should be the prerequisite for leadership in the New Permanent Golden Age.

3 - Visions Of A Golden Age

MAN'S DESTINY

It is part of our divine plan to grow, to evolve, to become more God-like, to use our creative abilities in the physical realm. We voluntarily chose embodiment in the physical realm. Nobody forced us to do so. Creation in this realm, which is of a lower vibratory level, is more difficult. The additional experience of embodiment will enable us to rise higher in our future state of development, after we have returned home to our I AM Presence, which all must do.

Man must learn who he is, must recognize that he is a creator, and as such must be master of what he creates. As a creator, he must consciously control his thoughts, words and actions, on a daily basis. Cosmic Law is a stern teacher, and the Law does not apply itself. All creation is a self-conocious effort, and if the individual upon whom this great gift of life has been bestowed refuses to take his respon-

sibility and to do his duty, his experiences will prod him with misery until he does. The progress of mankind is strictly determined by self-merit.

The Masters give assistance when allowed to do so, but They are not permitted to redeem the karma that follows the misuse of energy. It takes effort on the physical plane to bring the Masters into action. When mankind uses higher knowledge in a constructive way, the Masters are free to increase their assistance.

Perfection, dominion, harmonious use and control of all substance, is the Original Divine Blueprint for humanity. The attention to his source of life, to the giver of every good and perfect thing, is the "golden key" that opens the door.

Discord will cease in the outer experience of man through self-conscious effort in understanding Cosmic Law, God's Law, and in the realization that God is within every individual, and expressing His fullness through him. Man, himself, is the conscious director of his future activities. His destiny is to become a co-creator with God. The rate of progress towards this goal is strictly determined by self-merit.

A BLUEPRINT FOR A GOLDEN AGE

Having discussed our destiny and ultimate goal, let us now focus upon the reason we elected to embody upon the physical plane. We chose embodiment to become master of the energies and vibrations prevailing upon this plane, and to use that mastery to expand the kingdom of God in the physical realm. In other words, we chose this experience to utilize our God-given talents and abilities to create and manifest on the physical plane **One Nation under God.** Such an activity of accomplishment has been termed by the Masters as a "Golden Age."

As we understand from the previous chapters, there have been several Golden Ages in the past, and there is no reason that we cannot manifest such a Golden Age in the future. The plan of the Masters for bringing in such a Golden Age contains the following key elements:

1) There must be a clear concept of what a Golden Age encompasses. The ultimate goal and the overall framework of a Golden Age need to be defined so it can be clearly vizualized. This establishes the direction.
2) There must be a well-outlined plan of action. This plan of action needs to incorporate the ways and means of fulfilling the goal and of designating the vehicle needed to bring us to our avowed destination. The action plan also needs to define the functions of the coordinating center and the organizational network necessary to accomplish the goal. Finally, we need to talk about the qualifications required of the people who are to be the standard-bearers.

Re-establishing a Golden Age is no small task. It cannot be brought in overnight. Therefore, the model must contain intermediate and near-term goals, and these goals must be measurable, achievable and realistic. Then having set those goals, we must prepare a step-by-step action plan to implement the model.

One student asked me, "Considering what the Masters said about the current crisis the Earth is facing, is there time left at all to write books and to read them?" This was two years ago, and I told him then that I didn't know, but I surely would try to present the plan of the Masters for a Golden Age and a proposed plan of action to bring it about. Yes, I believe there is still time, but I also agree with the Masters that time is rapidly running out, and there is a need for the program to be carried out without delay.

Since we have the benefit of the detailed account of the Messengers Ballard and Innocenti, elaborating Saint Germain's and El Morya's plan to bring in a New Golden Age, I suggest we use that plan as our blueprint. In addition, the examples given by the Masters of mankind's life in the Garden of Eden, the Sahara Civilization, the civilization in Meru (South America) and on Poseidonis together with the description of the Golden Ages of Greece and Egypt should be considered.

Man was not make to work by the sweat of the brow. In some Atlantean periods, precipitation and levitation were the order of the day. During the time period called the "Garden of Eden," there was no veil, no barrier shutting down the visible presence of the Ascended Host. After the fall of man, there were time periods when the veil was rent, demonstrating that it can be done once more. Dominion over so-called matter and universal life-force are God-given attributes. These virtues will reappear in proportion to mankind's willingness to give up the lifestyle of the "pursuit of happiness." When man, instead of blaming some external foe, looks within himself, casts the beam from his own eye, and changes his habits, he achieves mastery over anything within himself that is not of God.

Temples need to be built where students can come from many parts of the globe to revitalize themselves and bathe in the purifying essence of the flame of the temple. The flames, themselves, are to be visible again, just as in early Atlantean times in the Temple of Archangel Zadkiel near today's Cuba.

Re-reading the account of the Sahara Civilization brings to mind several important ingredients of a Golden Age. At that time the King-Emperor was assisted by a council of fourteen Ascended Masters. The government consisted of seven departments, which controlled the activities of science, industry and art. Each department head worked directly with the council, and therefore was attuned at all times with the divine plan. Everybody served for the good of all. This example demonstrates the many-faceted character of a Golden Age. Perfection and harmonious control of energy need to be expressed in **all** of the seven channels of contructive expression, not just in the field of religion.

NEW AGE GROUP ACTIVITIES

Introduction

In 1952 the Ascended Masters Saint Germain and El Morya requested a cosmic service that would cover the entire planet. They reasoned that through such an endeavor not only the planetary crisis could be brought under control, but also a NEW Permanent Golden Age could be introduced. The vehicle for implementing such a plan was group activity. Therefore, the establishment of groups as a means of carrying out the design of the blueprint for a New Golden Age is the need of the hour.

According to their purpose, groups may include the following functions:

1) Religious Worship. Service to God and the Ascended Masters (decreeing, contemplation, music.)
2) Scientific Research. To do individual or group research and share the results. Projects selected are those which have the potential of hastening in the New Golden Age.
3) Doing other projects which serve the common good, giving emphasis that members of Ascended Master Teaching groups play an active role, making this planet a better place to live in. Examples are endeavors that result in:

a) better standards in the field of local, state and national government
b) better laws and law enforcement (such as review of the system by which people are taxed)
c) higher standards in journalism
d) improving the quality of existing TV and radio programs
e) harmonious and effective labor-management relationships, resulting in better consumer products. (Many agree that it was the concept of Quality Circles that is primarily responsible for the improvement of Japanese products.)

4) Individual Development.
a) Instructions on Cosmic Law
b) Meetings on spiritual healing
c) Discussions on topics of mutual interest

5) Meetings for young students.
a) Opportunity to meet other students, providing for relaxation and fun in an atmosphere of non-drinking and non-smoking.
b) Under the general guidance of adults to carry out some of the other functions mentioned above.

It is evident that there exists an almost limitless field of activity for students of Ascended Master Teaching, and each may express God's perfection and virtues in the physical realm, all according to his individual talents and promptings.

Religious Worship

In each two-thousand-year cycle, a religion is evolved by the Intelligences who represent the Godhead for this period. The religion takes into consideration the natural tendencies of those individuals who are to be the focal point of the message to be given and the requirements of the time.

As the Hierarchy of the Earth set into motion the two-thousand-year cycle of the Seventh Ray under the direction of Saint Germain, it introduced the type of religious worship which will become the predominant activity of the masses in the future.

The particular God-virtues of the Seventh Ray and of Saint Germain are uplifting ritual and ceremonial worship, expressed in group activity. In group activity, every participant who works in conscious cooperation with its director, becomes a focus of the virtues of the Seventh Ray, and a magnetizing center through his own heartbeat.

Let us proceed with the account of the Masters and define the responsibilities of the director and the remaining members of the group. The energy of the director directs and focuses the energies of the group. His task is to unify the consciousness of the group through invocations of the powers of the Sacred Fire, decreeing, **directed** visualizations, songs, keynotes of the Masters, and other uplifting musical compositions. The ability of the director to obtain and hold the interest of the group, as well as the joyous, willing cooperation of each member, determines the efficacy of the service. Energies that are released through a sense of "duty" or "fear" are practically useless in the Master's work. Joyous, happy energy is the hope of heaven.

The director must endeavor to give all members equal opportunity to serve and to express themselves. Some love to decree, some love to visualize, some participate happily in songs. It is better to have a fifteen-minute span of a certain activity and keep it "alive" than a much longer one if such strains the undeveloped bodies of the individuals. Ceremonial worship is the balanced use of the harmonious blend of the energies of the participants. It creates new causes for good, and dissolves those of an inharmonious nature.

Each group member should realize he/she is a member of a team and in order to go into a certain direction, all members must follow. The energies (thoughts and feelings) need to focused in the direction the group is going. Daydreaming, soaring off into a daze, form the ingredients for the weak link in a chain. Each member of the group should remember that within his own heart and the heart of others dwells the focalized Ray of the Presence and Power of the Godhead, containing within itself the pattern of his own future greatness, even as the seed of a flower contains within itself the pattern of the future flower.

Each individual must also realize, that individual development and mastery **must** proceed hand in hand with impersonal service. We call this service "impersonal" because we freely give of our energies and we do not know to what specific beneficial purpose these energies will be used by the Ascended Host. Giving freely and joyously of our energies, and directing these energies **consciously** to the Great Intelligences who form the focus of the Godhead on our Earth, is the prime purpose of the meeting. This enables the Masters to multiply that energy and use it for the benefit of the race.

When these meetings are held at regular intervals, a certain rhythmic pulse is set into motion, which results in the formation of a permanent magnetic forcefield above the sanctuary. The Masters can utilize this forcefield long after the meeting is over. A forcefield has the additional benefit of forming a canopy of protection for the group members and their general location.

In order to achieve the purpose of the meeting in a most effective manner, it is well to keep in mind the following:

1. The inner and physical bodies of the members of the group need to be quiet. This is achieved through musical compositions of a soothing and inspirational nature, enabling the present members of the Angelic Host to go into action and prepare the inner bodies of the students to receive the greatest possible blessings. Quieting the inner bodies also raises each individual to his own highest potential service to the group and to the Master Intelligence who is presiding and working with such a group.

2. The purification of the bodies and auras of the students, the director, and the surrounding atmosphere through the invocation of the Violet Flame.

3. Recognition of the God-Power focused through each participant, which is the authority by which energy is set into motion and directed toward ultimately good effects.

4. Acceptance of the Presence of — and access to — the Ascended Host of Light, the Angelic, Devic, Cherubic and Seraphic Hosts, as conscious co-workers in the activities of the group work.

When these requirements have been met, the Directing Intelligence of the Godhead, either through the God-Presence of the Director or an Ascended Master or Angelic Guest, will utilize the ritual to the greatest possible extent according to the requirements of the hour.

The Power of the Spoken Word- the Key

As shown previously in Part I, the activity of decreeing had a profound impact on the evolution of the race. The Ascended Master El Morya, referring to the Second Dispensation (The Bridge to Freedom) said flatly, that if it had not been for the decreeing, he would not have even bothered to apply for this dispensation. It was this activity that made it possible for the Earth to continue to keep its place in the galaxy during the tests and trials of the 1930's and 1950's, and it may be this activity of the students of today that will make it possible to continue having the Earth as a planetary home. Since decreeing is something new to the western consciousness, and since the Masters placed so much emphasis upon this activity, perhaps this subject should now be considered in more detail.

The activity of decreeing sets aside groups of Ascended Master Teaching from all other New Age groups. Praying is good, and so is meditation. They help the individual's spiritual growth. Both help to create a beautiful individual aura that may bless others, BUT THESE ACTIVITIES DO NOT HELP A MASTER! A Master, in order to give assistance to a group or an individual depends upon a return of energy that is voluntarily and consciously directed to him. Decreeing, contemplation (meditation coupled with the student's attention resting upon the Master), and songs incorporating the name and special activity of a Master, are the type of energy the Master can use. Of these, decreeing and songs are the most effective.

To further explain the necessity of decreeing, the Master El Morya said, "If you receive from the universal source an inbreath into your lungs, and you refuse to breathe out and give that breath back to the universe, seeking to hold it in your body, you bring about the destruction of your form. In the same manner, the energy released by the chela in impersonal service to Life brings a return of energy from above in added knowledge, in added understanding, in a momentum of healing, and in a momentum of supply. But if the energy given by a Master is not used for a humanitarian purpose, and if he were to release more, the lifestream would eventually pass on of spiritual surfeit in the same manner that the body would die of condensed breath."

A BALANCE MUST BE GIVEN FOR ANY ASSISTANCE WHICH WE RECEIVE FROM A MASTER. If the assistance is given in the form of new instruction, a certain amount of the energy must be consciously returned, in addition to sharing this information with other honest, earnest and sincere seekers of truth. This is a point many group leaders and chelas don't understand. IT IS IMPOSSIBLE FOR A Master to give out new information to a group, if the original message is not UTILIZED TO THE FULLEST EXTENT POSSIBLE, AND IF IT IS NOT SHARED WITH THE REMAINING PEOPLE IN THE WORLD!

Let me briefly summarize how decrees should be given:

1) Decree in a standing position. Become still, calm all bodies, and give your attention to the I AM Presence.

2) If possible, decree in groups. The more people there are, the more energy will be released. If one member daydreams, does not understand what's being said, or does not visualize what's being said, he then becomes the weak link in the chain. The entire group is less effective. Therefore, no one should be admitted to a decree group, unless he has at least some understanding of this teaching. The mere repetition of words is useless.

3) Since visualization is so important, and since the western consciousness has difficulty in concentrating on anything — watch yourself sometimes to see how many seconds you concentrate unwaveringly upon any one item — decreeing should be stopped as soon as anyone in the group becomes tired. As the group matures, the decree period can be gradually increased in length.

4) There needs to be a balanced control of energy put forward by each individual member. Some individuals can be extremely positive in the use of a low, masterful tone, conveying a strong feeling. Others

cannot convey feeling except by the exertion of a measure of physical force, resulting in a louder voice tone. Here, freedom is the order of the day.

5) The competency of the director in drawing the energy into a rhythmic beat determines the efficacy of the decree. This is exactly the principle followed in using a battering ram against a locked door. Through the misuse of energy during many previous embodiments there has been a build-up of negative energy which needs to be dislodged and transmuted. All this energy cannot be transmuted with one simple affirmation. Therefore the basis of the decree pattern is rhythm and repetition.

6) The tempo of decreeing is important. I have heard of one group in the United States decreeing so rapidly one could hardly understand what was being said. On the other hand, I heard two groups in Germany decree so slowly that there appeared to be no rhythm at all; it sounded more like affirmations or fiats. The answer lies somewhat between both extremes.

Decreeing on a rhythmic, periodic basis creates an energized forcefield. The Masters can use the energy from this forcefield even if the group is not in session.

Decrees lower the mental forms of visualizations into the condensed energy of the physical realm. Decree groups are the requirement of the hour.

The accumulation of mankind's misqualified energy throughout the ages awaits its transmution. With sufficient decree groups it is possible to minimize the destructive chaos that the Earth is facing now. It may even be possible to prevent the destruction entirely. But that must be done without delay!

Spiritual Healing

While in physical embodiment is appears that we are totally separate from God. This is not so! God is closer than our breath. Regardless of what the evidence may show, we, as individuals in physical embodiment, are still connected to our I AM Presence, which is anchored in our heart. The son (the I AM Presence) has not, and never will, lose his connection to the Father (Helios and Vesta, the creator of the spiritual garments), and the Holy Spirit (Alpha and Omega, the supplier of life-energy for this galaxy.)

Before the fall of man there was visual contact with God's helpers, the Ascended Host. We must look with the inner eye, become still, and follow the guiding light, the still, small voice from within. Our I AM Presence, our connection to the Sun and the Great Central Sun, (which represents God as closely as we can comprehend Him) is our ever-present help in times of distress, during the appearance of illness, during a period of poor financial supply, or the lack of any good thing. In addition, we can call on the help of the Ascended Host. This is our God-given privilege! Therefore, physical embodiment should not prevent us from demonstrating perfection. As a matter of fact, it gives us opportunity to do so.

Any disharmonious experience should be viewed with the lens of the inner eye, looking beyond the testimony of the five outer senses. It should be recognized that God is not the dispenser of sin, sickness and death, but the giver of every perfect gift. It should be realized that imperfect conditions occur only through incorrect, disharmonious use of energy by the individual himself, and that each individual can contribute towards reversing the situation, by right and constructive use of energy.

This energy may be used in healing the sick. Students of this teaching are taught how this is done. One can still himself and call the Mighty I AM Presence into action, making it the only authority over the discordant condition.

Then we call on a Master who specializes in healing and mercy (Mary, Archangel Raphael, Jesus, Nada, Hilarion, Kwan Yin). This is followed by calling on the Law of Forgiveness and by using the Violet Flame. We can call to Mighty Astrea to remove the causes and cores of the discordant condition. In addition, we can visualize the healing presence of one of the above Masters (the countenances of about 15 Masters are known), and we can play the music containing the keynote of the particular Master involved.

This is not wishful thinking. We are talking about Truth, a mighty reality! It has been estimated that altogether, over 20,000 people attending Mr. Ballard's lectures were healed.

Physical embodiment serves a vital purpose. It is a needed experience for those brave souls who chose it as a means of gaining higher levels of accomplishment. Gaining mastery on the physical plane enables individuals to grow spiritually. Physical embodiment and experience on the physical plane demands a physical body.

As we come closer to God, the rate of vibration of our physical body will be accelerated, and its beauty, purity, and perfection will once more become manifest.

The Master Hilarion is assisting doctors, constantly finding new ways to improve the healing process. This can be seen as an act of mercy for the benefit of those who do not manifest the type of consciousness, which permits spiritual healing.

There needs to be a recognition that both methods of healing, physical and spiritual are appropriate, depending upon the level of consciousness and other conditions involved. Physicians need to understand that the physical body is only one of seven bodies, and others need to understand that the medical profession is very much needed under today's conditions. In the Golden Age, a cooperation and better understanding of physicians and spiritual healers is necessary.

Research

It is the goal of the Ascended Master Hilarion and the Brotherhood of Truth to draw the interest and cooperation of the scientifically-minded lifestreams of the Earth and teach them the exact science, as used by the Creator. Each individual of the Brotherhood is committed to a relentless quest for truth, a never-ending task. Individuals expressing the virtues of the Ray of Truth and Science (the fifth ray) are urged to share this newly-found pearl of great price with others, so they may also partake of this wisdom. Therefore it should be one of the functions of Ascended Master Teaching groups to perform scientific research including the ancient history of man and to engage in other projects that benefit the progress of the race. Finding artifacts attesting to Shamballa, the Meru Civilization, and the Sahara Civilization would be valuable, indeed. Then there are the remains of Atlantean temples and cities buried at the bottom of the Atlantic to uncover.

The Masters of Wisdom said that many inventions have been readied, waiting for a receptive consciousness for manifestation in the outer world. But to gain more information, we must first make good use of what we already know. This way we give a balance; it enables us to receive more.

One of the things which could be researched, are the ancient power boxes. According to the Masters the wisdom and technology during Atlantean Ages surpassed the accomplishments of modern technology in many areas. Universal energy, contained in the surrounding atmosphere, was harnessed for lighting, heating and propulsion of vehicles. It was stored and transmitted through power boxes. The Masters said that this accomplishment shall be achieved again.

There are now many individual researchers doing work along non-orthodox, unconventional lines, sensing this is the only way to obtain true answers. There is much duplication of effort and there needs to be direction at the local, national, and international level. This points out the need for research centers which serve to collect and store important data. In addition, these centers could do research of their own, act as a clearinghouse of ideas, and bring like-minded individuals together.

During some of the prior ages there were research centers where religious scientists worked, testing and applying the laws of nature for mankind's benefit. There is no reason that this cannot be repeated today. Why is it, that religion and science are often portrayed as irreconcilable opposites? Without the inner values, which only true religion can bestow, scientific research fails to acknowledge the universal fount of creation. This could easily lead to materialism and a denial of God.

There is some indication that the Masters of Wisdom intended to establish a research center as part of the Second New Age Dispensation. The Maha Chohan said in September, 1954: "When I am enabled through the limited karma of those who choose to so avail themselves to create a permanent research center, I can in good conscience release the activities of the Sacred Fire which, if applied and drawn through the energies of those participating, will be all the proof that is required of the efficacy of the practical application of the Law. Those incorporating the truths given in the energies of their own bodies will then be well prepared to carry that truth into the world of form.

This was our original design. Through the clamoring of the outer self and through the intrusion of many wills, we have seemingly deviated somewhat from our original purpose. We shall endeavor in the future however, to again draw forth that concentrated energy and draw around Ourselves, lifestreams capable of receiving — capable of offering their energies, to hold a harmonious sphere of influence long enough for the presence of the Master to convey not only the word, but also the feeling, and, allowing it to enter into the consciousness of the chelas, make a workable and practical pattern whereby the miracles and marvels spoken of will become fact.

The creation of a spiritual forcefield for a research center such as we had on Atlantis and on Lemuria become the obligation of every member of such a community, and the sustaining of that forcefield without a flicker of vibratory action of discord or disharmony becomes the responsibility and obligation of each one, through mastery and control of his own energies. Besides the research and the drawing forth of the spiritual law, we must have a practical laboratory where the law is put into action."

Once a research project has been completed, there must be unbiased reporting. The findings must be objectively stated, regardless of whether or not they fit into an existing pattern or theory. It should be remembered that the ray of science is also the ray of truth.

We must press on in our search into **all** facets of life. To the true religious scientist and researcher there is never an end; there is always another step toward greater heights and larger measures of accomplishment. Recognizing God and His laws, as they apply to our sphere of activity, is the work of eternity.

CO-WORKERS NEEDED

According to the Ascended Masters, a cosmic service is required that covers the entire planet. In this way the current crisis can be brought under control. The students of Ascended Master Teaching must unite their strength and join their energies to more effectively stem the tide of evil that must be rooted out of the human race before the permanent age of peace and world brotherhood can be established. Reading this book or others should be just the very beginning. It provides much knowledge, but what is learned must be put into practice. It is just the first step in a journey of a thousand miles.

All of us at some time contributed toward the problems the Earth is facing now. Jointly we fell, jointly it is our responsibility to get the Earth out of the present dilemma, and restore the harmony, beauty and perfection of the Garden of Eden.

Is it not a magnificent opportunity for us to reach those blessed individuals who perhaps all of their life had some inner urging "that there was more," and who for some reason or another never had a chance to be exposed to this teaching?

Serving God and the Masters gives one a magnificent opportunity to give a balance to life. The Law of Life, the law of one's being, is impersonal service.

Let us resolve to serve the Great White Brotherhood NOW! There is such a thing as quality of consciousness, this is most important, but there is also such a thing as strength in numbers.

On this subject, the Masters said the following:

"Those whose studies and convictions have given them a clearer and deeper insight into the causes acting behind the present manifestations of world chaos need to put aside their separate interests and individual prides, and meet together on a common ground, presenting a united front to the small minority of misguided humanity who are responsible for the menace of communism and war.

Less than 1% of mankind are responsible for the major distresses that burden the great majority of the people. Their unpleasant strength lies in the unity of their energies, endeavors and disintegrating purpose."

"At this time we are seeking those who are willing to be conscious co-workers with the Spiritual Hierarchy."

"It has been said 'One with God is a majority' and that is an eternal truth. One man's vision brought the Santa Maria across the Atlantic! One man's vision established a free America! ONE intelligence, God directed, has more than once saved this planet from dissolution! This person held the connection between the human and the divine! Just preceding the coming of Sanat Kumara there remained four lifestreams who held this connection. Four individuals out of ten billion, and yet it was enough."

The Eloah of Peace said, "Whatever you wish to accomplish that amounts to anything, requires the dedication of your life!"

Another Master said in the 1950's, "It is admitted many of you decree for world peace, but the intensity of the decrees and the number of those engaged in this activity is insufficient. **The nations of the Earth are sitting on a powder keg.** Beloved students, so are you! It is your responsibility, your duty, as part of balancing your account with the Cosmic Law to serve the Light! I not only ask and urge you, but I say with all authority, it is your duty to help now. Your future spiritual development depends on this decision. The service that we wish you to do, is needed NOW!"

"Your mission is similar to mine. Before I came into the world of form, I was charged with a mission, that is, to manifest unto all mankind the full perfection of our Father. You were also so charged when you were created! (March 1956, Jesus)

"There were some 300 million lifestreams who were passed by the Karmic Board in the 1950's, all of whom have vowed to serve the light according to their capacity."

"At the other side millions are begging to come into embodiment and you (students), who have physical vehicles, must become more and more cognizant of the magnificent opportunity that is before you."

"All of you did contribute at some time towards the problems the Earth is facing now. Therefore it is your responsibility and duty to help to get the Earth out of its present dilemma."

"The substance of the Earth has been destructively qualified by human discordant feeling. What do you think it would mean if mankind failed to come back into the Light? It would mean second death for millions of humanity."

"People who have the karma that goes back to the Lemurian ages, the ages on Atlantis, Babylon, and Greece, had their four lower bodies rebuilded for one purpose, to bring to the Earth the knowledge of the Golden Age. Then having accepted that gift of grace they do not accept or spread that word of freedom to others. Think of the karma that soul shall meet when it stands before the Judgment Board."

"One day, as the veil thins, with your physical sight, you may see the members of the inner kingdom; it will be then a joy to work with them in bringing to fruition the Golden Age."

"In the days that are to come, we require an Army of Light ALL OVER THIS EARTH, of individuals in a constant state of alertness, a constant state of grace, a constant state of harmony, balance and poise, ready to move at an instant! Then, if an activity is about to take place, and we desire to direct a thousand light-rays simultaneously, a thousand leaders will stand and a thousand groups will go into action and disaster will be averted. This is the training for the few who walk under the banner of freedom in My name." (Saint Germain, 1961)

A PROPOSED PLAN OF ACTION

Once again a magnetizing center for a new Christ-message is needed. The Masters have said they are preparing a new Avatar who is waiting for the proper moment to embody (dictation of the 1950's). Thanks to the mercy of the God, the pure Ascended Master message, which comes like the dove, humbly, simply, and unadorned, may again be given to mankind.

How can the dispensation necessary for this to happen be granted, if the message of the last two dispensations has not been fully utilized? How can the new message be brought forth, when in spite of the repeated plea of the Masters, a great part of the original dictations is either not published, not translated, or is not freely available? In addition I am not aware of any existing organization that limits its teachings to the original message of the Masters as given through Mr. Ballard and G. Innocenti; and that is designed and structured to provide the global service asked for.

Therefore, a new effort is required to re-introduce and disseminate the meaning of the original message. A NEW BRIDGE, a new link, a connection over which the counsel of the Ascended Masters may reach the intellect of the outer consciousness is very much needed. It is up to a few enlightened individuals to build such a bridge, using as a pattern the original blueprint designed by Saint Germain and El Morya.

This bridge must be a structure of light-energy woven by the students on one side, and by the responding energies of the Masters of Wisdom on the other. Once this vital connection is completed, and firmly anchored by students, a direct link between one or more individuals residing on the physical realm with the Ascended Masters on their realm can once more be formed. When this forcefield has been given sufficient love and dedication by the students, no force in the world can stop the loving, tangible counsel of the Great Ones, and a new flow of information may be given. Then a new messenger can bring the requirement of the hour to the consciousness of the people. Once the message freely flows through the messenger, it must be translated into every language and spread to every corner of the globe. This is not fanciful thinking, this is reasoning based on the rules of unerring Cosmic Law!

Starting anew seems like an unsurmountable task. However, until there is a new messenger or avatar, there are thousands of pages of the original dictations. The Masters commented that the knowledge released was ten times more than is needed for our ascension. More knowledge was given than we can ever hope to apply in a lifetime. In addition to the information given in this book, there are the publications by A.D.K. Luk, such as *Law of Life* (two volumes), *Law of Life and Teachings by Divine Beings* (three volumes), a publication on group activity, and decree books that can be recommended to students. The first three books of the Saint Germain Foundation, originally published in the 1930's, have been available in bookstores since 1983.

Fortunately, it does not take many individuals to serve as torchbearers, the heralds of the New Age. Quality of consciousness, and a firm determination to serve the Masters, are of prime importance. These qualities, even though exhibited by only a few, are more important than previous experience. Both the dispensations of the 1930's and 1950's were started by less than a handful of people.

The type of group activity mentioned in the previous chapter is required NOW. The energy spent on the physical plane in the initial effort will be amplified by the Masters of Wisdom, and will help build a strong bridge of light-energy leading to the Divine Realm. All this energy directed in the right channels will make it possible for the guardians of the race to give additional information in the future.

Over the course of the years, there has been a persistent effort by various individuals to personally influence and change this teaching. This will require the constant vigilance of the students. If given loving attention and if it is guarded well, Saint Germain's effort will prosper.

Volunteers are needed now to bring the plan of the Ascended Masters into fruition. The first phase of this effort will consist of bringing people together who wish to actively participate in this holy mission and do the necessary preparatory work for the global service that is required.

Two and one-half million years ago, thirty individuals from all part of the globe gathered on the shores of the Gobi-Sea. Many had had a wearisome journey. Some had to cross many continents and oceans. A burning desire lighted their way, the imprint on their etheric bodies of a shining city, later called Shamballa. After arriving upon the shore of the Gobi-Sea, the strongest of the pilgrims brought forth their vision, and it was confirmed in the hearts of others.

Building a new Shamballa is a distinct possibility. It will depend on the efforts of the Ascended Master students of today.

Bibliography, Part III

Cayce, E.E. *Cayce on Atlantis.* New York, Castle Books, 1968

Donnelly, S. *Atlantis the Antediluvian World.* Blauvelt, New York, Rudolf Steiner Publications

Fell, B. *America B.C.* New York, Pocket Books, 1976

Luk, A.D.K. *Law of Life Enlightener.* Bi-monthly magazine. Oklahoma City, 1124 N. Meta Ave., A.D.K. Luk Publications, 1983

Luk, A.D.K. *Law of Life,* Vol. I & II. Oklahoma City, 1124 N. Meta Ave., A.D.K. Luk Publications, 1959 & 1960

Montgomery, R. *The World Before.* New York, Coward, McCann & Geoghegan, 1976

Printz, T. *The Bridge to Freedom.* Monthly Journal. Kings Park, New York, The Bridge to Freedom, 1952 through 1961*

Rehwinkel, A.M. *The Flood.* Saint Louis

Schmidt, F. *Mitteilungen Des Eremiten (Explanations of a Hermit).* Mount Shasta, California 96067, P.O. Box 466, Ascended Master Teaching Foundation, 1982

Schmidt, F. *Kundgebungen des Eremiten* (Messages of a Hermit).* Cleveland, Ohio, Felix Schmidt, 1951

Steiger, B. *Atlantis Rising.* New York, Dell Publishing Co., 1973

* No longer published (as of 1983)

FOR NEW PRICES
SEND FOR BOOKLIST

BOOKS DISTRIBUTED BY AMTF

MAN, HIS ORIGIN, HISTORY AND DESTINY by W. Schroeder, 336 pp. Using a variety of sources, this new title presents mankind's unrecorded history. Much of the material has not been researched before, and it has not been available to the general public. Written in chronological order, the reader learns of the conditions prevailing during the advent of man on Earth, including his origin and his age. Fascinating highlights of the Lemurian and Atlantean civilizations are given. Also depicted are accounts of the unchronicled history of Jesus and the oracles of Delphi. Practical solutions are presented to meet today's planetary crisis. $10.00

UNVEILED MYSTERIES by Godfre Ray King, 288 pp. This book contains Mr. Ballard's group of first experiences, following his meeting with the Ascended Master Saint Germain on Mount Shasta. We are happy to present to the students a full, unabridged copy of this priceless book, which heralded in the New Age.$9.75

THE FIRST RAY by the Ascended Master El Morya, 128 pp. Herein are described the God-Virtues of the First Ray, how the dispensation for the "Bridge to Freedom" was obtained, and the purpose of this endeavor. In the section "The Spiritual Caravan" El Morya extends an invitation to students to join him in a global effort, bringing in a New Golden Age. $5.75

THE SEVEN MIGHTLY ELOHIM SPEAK ON THE SEVEN STEPS TO PRECIPITATION by Thomas Printz, 256 pp. This book contains the original account of the principles employed in the creation of our planet by the Builders of the Universe, known as the Seven Elohim. The principles of precipitation are part of the eternal Law of Life. Therefore man, as Co-Creator with God, may utilize them to his advantage in his daily affairs. $9.45

THE SEVENTH RAY by the Ascended Master Saint Germain, 128 pp. This book consists of several addresses by Saint Germain. Featured are primal requirements for an efficacious service, and the responsibilities of each group member, including its leader. An indispensable aid for those involved in group activities. $5.75

MEMOIRS OF BELOVED MARY, MOTHER OF JESUS by Thomas Printz, 192 pp. Chronicled here are several addresses by Mary, depicting details of her last embodiment, with Jesus. Many of these are not given in the Bible, such as early life experiences of Jesus, his trip to India, and details of his ascension. The reader learns of Mary's journey to Europe, including her travels to Fatima, Lourdes and Glastonbury. $8.00

For additional titles send for book list.

ORDERING INFORMATION

Write to AMTF P.O. Box 466, Mount Shasta, CA 96067. Delivery Charges, US: $2.50 first book, additional books - $0.50/copy. Outside US: $3.00 first book, additional books -$1.00/copy. Sales tax 6%, California residents only.